EXPLORING NEW HORIZONS IN OBSTETRICS AND GYNECOLOGY

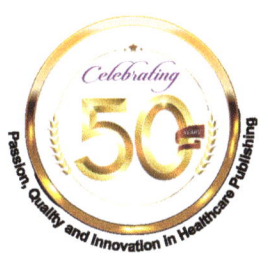

EXPLORING NEW HORIZONS IN OBSTETRICS AND GYNECOLOGY
(WHAT TO DO NEXT AFTER MD IN OBSTETRICS AND GYNECOLOGY?)

Editors

Aswath Kumar R
MD FICOG
Diploma in Advanced Laparoscopy (France)
Diploma in Laparoscopic Management of
Advanced Endometriosis (Austria)
Fellow (Gynec-Oncology)
The Gujarat Cancer and Research Institute
(GCRI), Ahmedabad, Gujarat
Professor
Department of Gynecology
Jubilee Mission Medical College
Thrissur, Kerala, India
FOGSI Quiz Committee Chairperson
(2012–2015)
Vice President, FOGSI, 2019
Vice President, KFOG, 2017

Nilesh Balkawade
MS DNB MNMAS FIAGE
Fellow, Reproductive Medicine
Consultant, IVF and Endoscopy,
Indira IVF, Pune, Maharashtra
Ex-Assistant Professor
Department of Obstetrics and
Gynecology
Dr DY Patil Medical College,
Pune, Maharashtra, India
National Coordinator
FOGSI Quiz Committee (2018–2020)
Jt Treasurer, POGS (2015–2016)

Co-Editors

S Shantha Kumari
MD DNB FICOG FRCPI (Ireland)
FRCOG (UK)
Chairperson, ICOG, 2018
Consultant, Yashoda Hospital
Hyderabad, Telangana, India
ICOG Secretary (2015–2017)
Member, FIGO Working Group
(on Violence Against Women)
Vice President, FOGSI 2013

Tushar Kar
MD MICOG FICOG FICMCH
Fellowship Laparoscopic Surgery (USA)
Department of Obstetrics and
Gynecology
SCB Medical College
Cuttack, Odisha, India
Chairperson, ICOG (2019–2020)
Vice President, FOGSI (2010–2011)
Chairperson, Oncology, FOGSI (2004–2009)

Parag Biniwale
MD FICOG FICMCH
Consultant Obstetrician and Gynecologist
Pune, Maharashtra, India
Secretary, ICOG

Foreword
Nandita Palshetkar

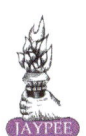

JAYPEE BROTHERS MEDICAL PUBLISHERS
The Health Sciences Publisher
New Delhi | London | Panama

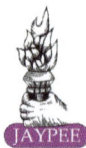 **Jaypee Brothers Medical Publishers (P) Ltd**

Headquarters
Jaypee Brothers Medical Publishers (P) Ltd
4838/24, Ansari Road, Daryaganj
New Delhi 110 002, India
Phone: +91-11-43574357
Fax: +91-11-43574314
Email: jaypee@jaypeebrothers.com

Overseas Offices

J.P. Medical Ltd
83 Victoria Street, London
SW1H 0HW (UK)
Phone: +44 20 3170 8910
Fax: +44 (0)20 3008 6180
Email: info@jpmedpub.com

Jaypee-Highlights Medical Publishers Inc
City of Knowledge, Bld. 235, 2nd Floor
Clayton, Panama City, Panama
Phone: +1 507-301-0496
Fax: +1 507-301-0499
Email: cservice@jphmedical.com

Jaypee Brothers Medical Publishers (P) Ltd
Bhotahity, Kathmandu, Nepal
Phone: +977-9741283608
Email: kathmandu@jaypeebrothers.com

Website: www.jaypeebrothers.com
Website: www.jaypeedigital.com

© 2019, Jaypee Brothers Medical Publishers

The views and opinions expressed in this book are solely those of the original contributor(s)/author(s) and do not necessarily represent those of editor(s) of the book.

All rights reserved. No part of this publication may be reproduced, stored or transmitted in any form or by any means, electronic, mechanical, photocopying, recording or otherwise, without the prior permission in writing of the publishers.

All brand names and product names used in this book are trade names, service marks, trademarks or registered trademarks of their respective owners. The publisher is not associated with any product or vendor mentioned in this book.

Medical knowledge and practice change constantly. This book is designed to provide accurate, authoritative information about the subject matter in question. However, readers are advised to check the most current information available on procedures included and check information from the manufacturer of each product to be administered, to verify the recommended dose, formula, method and duration of administration, adverse effects and contraindications. It is the responsibility of the practitioner to take all appropriate safety precautions. Neither the publisher nor the author(s)/editor(s) assume any liability for any injury and/or damage to persons or property arising from or related to use of material in this book.

This book is sold on the understanding that the publisher is not engaged in providing professional medical services. If such advice or services are required, the services of a competent medical professional should be sought.

Every effort has been made where necessary to contact holders of copyright to obtain permission to reproduce copyright material. If any have been inadvertently overlooked, the publisher will be pleased to make the necessary arrangements at the first opportunity. The **CD/DVD-ROM** (if any) provided in the sealed envelope with this book is complimentary and free of cost. **Not meant for sale.**

Inquiries for bulk sales may be solicited at: jaypee@jaypeebrothers.com

Exploring New Horizons in Obstetrics and Gynecology
(What to do next after MD in Obstetrics and Gynecology?)

First Edition: **2019**

ISBN: 978-93-5270-8291

Dedicated to

All Postgraduate Students and Consultants.

Contributors

Ajay Rane MBBS MSc MD FRCS FRCOG FRANZCOG CU FICOG (Hon) PhD FRCPI (Hon)
Professor and Head
Department of Obstetrics and Gynecology
Consultant Urogynecologist
James Cook University, Townsville
FIGO Fistula Chair
Board Member
Townsville Hospital and Health Service
Townsville, Australia

Anay Bhalerao MBBS MBA
Content Lead, the Asian Parent Community
Community: Tickled Media Pvt Ltd

Aparna N MCh
Resident
Department of Reproductive Medicine and Surgery
Amrita Institute of Medical Sciences
Kochi, Kerala, India

Aswath Kumar R MD FICOG
Diploma in Advanced Laparoscopy (France)
Diploma in Laparoscopic Management of Advanced Endometriosis (Austria)
Fellow (Gynec-Oncology)
The Gujarat Cancer and Research Institute (GCRI), Ahmedabad, Gujarat
Professor
Department of Gynecology
Jubilee Mission Medical College
Thrissur, Kerala, India
FOGSI Quiz Committee Chairperson (2012–2015)
Vice President, FOGSI, 2019
Vice President, KFOG, 2017

Deepa Ganesh
MBBS MS FMAS DMAS FICRS FIMA Dip MIS (Germany) Dip ALS (France) Dip ACG (USA) FIMSA
Director
DG Laser and Cosmetic Gynecology Clinic, Chennai, Tamil Nadu
Consultant, Laparoscopic
Robotic and Cosmetic Gynecologist
Lifeline/Apollo/Medway/SIMS Hospitals/Pearl Aesthetics
Chennai, Tamil Nadu, India

Fessy Louis T
Senior Consultant
Department of Reproductive Medicine and Surgery
Amrita Institute of Medical Sciences
Kochi, Kerala, India

Jiteeka Thakkar DGO DFP
IVF Consultant
Bloom IVF
MOGS Youth Council Member 2018–2019

Kajal Parikh
MBBS MS-OBGYN, FMAS (MUHS)
Jupiter Hospital (Thane), Thunga Hospital (Malad)
Mumbai, Maharashtra

K Subash Mallya DGO DNB MNAMS
Diploma in Gynec-Endoscopy (Germany)
PGDMLS
Consultant Gynecologist and Minimal Access Surgeon
PVS Hospital
Kozhikode, Kerala, India

Manish Machave
MD DNB (OB/GYN) MNAMS FICOG LLB
Diploma in Endoscopy (Germany)
Advanced Diploma in Gynecologic
Endoscopy (France)
Consultant, OB/GYN, Pune
Medicolegal Consultant

Megha Jayprakash MS DGO MRCOG
Associate Professor
Department of Obstetrics and Gynecology
Government Medical College
Thrissur, Kerala, India
Pursuing Fellowship in Gynecologic
Oncology in UK

Nilesh Balkawade
MS DNB MNMAS FIAGE
Fellow, Reproductive Medicine
Consultant, IVF and Endoscopy,
Indira IVF, Pune, Maharashtra
Ex-Assistant Professor
Department of Obstetrics and Gynecology
Dr DY Patil Medical College,
Pune, Maharashtra, India
National Coordinator
FOGSI Quiz Committee (2018–2020)
Jt Treasurer, POGS (2015–2016)

Rajendra Shitole MBBS DGO DNB
DMAS FMAS MNAMS Certificate in Robotic
Surgery
Consultant Obstetrician and Gynecologist
Laparoscopic and Robotic Surgeon
Assistant Professor
Dr DY Patil Medical College Hospital
and Research Centre
Pune, Maharashtra, India

Ramesh P MCh
Resident
Department of Reproductive Medicine
and Surgery
Amrita Institute of Medical Sciences
Kochi, Kerala, India

Raymond George MBBS MD
Maternal Fetal Medicine Specialist
Consultant
Department of Obstetrics and Gynecology
Rajagiri Hospital
Aluva, Kerala, India

Rohan Palshetkar MS OB/GYN
Assistant Professor
DY Patil School of Medicine
Managing Committee Member of
Maharashtra Chapter of ISAR, 2018–2020
MOGS Youth Council Member
2018–2019

Sandip Datta Roy
MBBS MS (OB/GYN)FICMCH FICS FMIS
(Fellowship in Gyneco-logical Endoscopy,
RGHUS, Bangalore)
Consultant Gynecologist
Laparoscopic Surgeon and Infertility
Specialist
Thrissur, Kerala, India

Santhosh Kuriakose
MBBS DGO MS (OB/GYN) Fellowship in
Gynecologic Oncology
In-Charge
Gynecologic Oncology Division
Department of Obstetrics and Gynecology
Government Medical College, Kozhikode
Chairman of Oncology Committee, KFOG
Kozhikode, Kerala, India

Sarveshwar Bhure MBBS
(BJ Medical College, Pune)
IAS (2010 Batch), Mission Director
National Health Mission
Director, Health and Family Welfare
(Additional Charge)
Government of Chhattisgarh

Shailesh Balkawade BE (Mech)
IPS (2009 Batch)
Superintendent of Police
Gadchiroli, Maharashtra, India

Tanvir MBBS MS (OB/GYN)
Diploma in Gynecological Endoscopy
Certificate of Specialist Accreditation PDCR
Consultant
Tanvir Hospital
Hyderabad, Telangana, India

Tushar Kar MD MICOG FICOG FICMCH
Fellowship Laparoscopic Surgery (USA)
Department of Obstetrics and
Gynecology
SCB Medical College
Cuttack, Odisha, India
Chairperson, ICOG (2019–2020)
Vice President, FOGSI (2010–2011)
Chairperson, Oncology, FOGSI (2004–2009)

Varsha Dange
MBBS DGO PG (Diploma in Health and
Hospital Management)
(PG Diploma in Medico-Legal Studies)
RCHO (Medical Department)
Pimpri-Chinchwad Municipal
Corporation, Pune
Contributor in RCH and
Family Welfare

Vivek Krishnan
Clinical Associate Professor and Head
Department of Fetal Medicine and
Perinatology
Amrita Institute of
Medical Sciences
Kochi, Kerala, India

Foreword

Dear Readers,

Greetings from the FOGSI President and her team!

Youngsters today are poised on the cusp of a technological revolution. With the easy availability of mobile networks and internet accessibility, scientific and educational materials in print and online, video courses, discussion forums, training workshops and programs being regularly conducted nationally and overseas, there is no dearth of high quality materials in the quest for updated knowledge.

The scenario today is much different from two or three decades ago when quality training and accessibility to such courses was limited and highly sought after. However, the entire gamut of options available to young trainees today can be overwhelming and confusing. After completion of postgraduation, there are so many options available currently that it is difficult to summarize and weigh the risks, benefits, and long-term viability of the different paths that one can take.

"Believe in yourself. Have faith in your abilities. Without a humble but reasonable confidence in your own powers you cannot be successful or happy"—Norman Vincent Peale

This excellent compendium is an attempt to provide a precise and detailed outline of the many options available to young gynecologists after they complete their postgraduation. Dr Aswath Kumar R, Vice President FOGSI, is a dynamic, hardworking and enthusiastic teacher who has trained several young gynecologists in endoscopic surgery and other allied branches of our specialty.

This book is his brainchild and he has worked hard along with his co-authors to provide the latest information to today's trainees, including fellowship courses, short diplomas, international traveling courses, and superspecialty training, among others. There is no similar text available in India, as of today!

I have no doubt that this book will go a long way toward helping young doctors make informed career choices, guide them regarding available courses and help to plan their future with a particular subspecialty in mind.

I wish the readers all the very best for their future, hope they join FOGSI, become committed *FOGSIans* and strengthen this amazing organization!

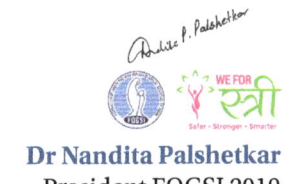

Dr Nandita Palshetkar
President FOGSI 2019

Preface

Obstetrics and Gynecology is a constantly evolving field! New things and innovations are coming up fast. So are options of what to do after MD gynecology!

It is not just the superspecialty, but also the varied branches which are attracting the Gen Next!

We could hardly imagine doctors as business administrators or entrepreneurs few decades ago! But things are changing rapidly! Doctors are seen to be successful in many walks of life. Be it their own field such as endoscopy or completely newer ones such as Law or MBA!! Life has taken a 360° turn when it comes to choosing professional course.

Some fields, although a part of Obstetrics and Gynecology, have now grown into huge superspecialty. Endoscopy, robotics and reproductive medicine has grown as a specialty field in Obstetrics and Gynecology. Cosmetic gynecology has just started to spread its wings and occupy the horizon. Public health is an old branch but is now being rejuvenated.

Civil services or MBA or international dimensions are few of the new horizons left to explore!

More is yet to come! You may be contended with yourself as an obstetrician or may be not!

Always remember that your present situation is not your final destination; the *Best is yet to come!!!*

We do not say that this book provides you with all options to look for after doing your MD/MS. But certainly, it will give you the right food for thoughts while thinking of, *"What to do next?"*

You have to think out of the box to be a successful person.

William Faulkner has rightly said,

You cannot Swim for new Horizons until
you have courage to Loose Sight of the Shore

Acknowledgments

We sincerely thank our postgraduate students for showing the faith in us and asking us the million dollar question, "What to do after MD?"

This made us to think about all options we could explore…Some were practical and are included here. Some might not be included in this first edition. Sky is the only limit when it comes to FLYING!

We thank our families for giving us that much needed energy in our wings, so that we can fly high, explore new horizons and bring some glimpses to you in form of this book.

We thank all our mentors, friends and seniors at FOGSI who helped us achieve different milestones in our lives.

We are thankful to M/s Jaypee Brothers Medical Publishers (P) Ltd, India, for bringing out this book wonderfully well.

Last but not the least, we thank all our teachers who have showed us the right path throughout our lives!!

Contents

1. Exploring New Horizons 1
   Aswath Kumar R, Nilesh Balkawade

2. Gynecological Endoscopy Training in India 6
   Sandip Datta Roy

3. Minimal Invasive Surgery (International) 24
   K Subash Mallya

4. Robotic Surgery: Next Frontier in
   Minimal Invasive Surgery 30
   Rajendra P Shitole

5. Gynecological Oncology 36
   Santhosh Kuriakose

6. Fetal Medicine 42
   Vivek Krishnan

7. High-risk Pregnancy and Perinatology 53
   Raymond George

8. MCh (Reproductive Medicine and Surgery) 57
   Fessy Louis T, Aparna N, Ramesh P

9. Fellowship in Reproductive Medicine and Surgery 64
   Rohan Palshetkar, Jiteeka Thakkar

10. Urogynecology Fellowship 71
    Tanvir, Ajay Rane

11. Public Health Sector and Family Planning 80
    Varsha Dange

12. MRCOG: A Roadmap 87
    Megha Jayprakash

13. USMLE and Future Prospects 99
    Kajal Parikh

14. Cosmetic Gynecology: An Overview 110
    Deepa Ganesh

15. **Civil Services (IAS/IPS)** 117
    Sarveshwar Bhure, Shailesh Balkawade

16. **Master of Business Administration: New Dimension** 123
    Anay Bhalerao

17. **Law Study: An Indispensable and Essential Action
    (Legum Baccalaureus: Condicio Sine Qua Non)** 128
    Manish Y Machave

18. **MICOG–MRCOG Course** 133
    Tushar Kar

Index *135*

CHAPTER 1

Exploring New Horizons

Aswath Kumar R, Nilesh Balkawade

"One Book, one Pen and one Teacher can change the world."
We all want to be successful in some forms or the other! We all have ambitions for the same! Some want to earn a "name", some want to earn "fame", some want to live a peaceful family life while some want to work day and night for the wellbeing of the Society!

"Intelligence without ambitions is a bird without wings."
Certainly it is not at all a bad thing to be ambitious! And one thing is not better than the other. Each individual is different hence his/her aspirations might differ. So it would not be right to say who is superior to whom while choosing the way of life.

A person who knows how to always have a job, but the person who knows "why" will always be his boss. Successful people solve problems, they never lack ideas that can build an organization, and they always have hope for a better future.

Steve Jobs has said, "Your time is limited, so don't waste it living someone else's life (Fig. 1.1)."

To be successful, you have to shed off your laziness, grab yourself together, prioritize things, set yourself specific goal(s), read and read voraciously,

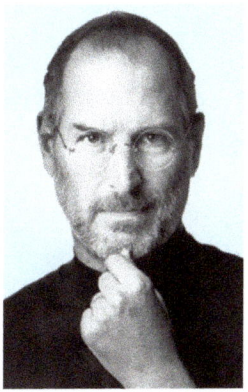

Fig. 1.1: Steve Jobs.

maintain the balance in work and personal life, prepare and persevere, give time to think and most importantly "act".

In the wise words of Tyrion Lannister, "A mind needs books like a sword needs a whetstone."

This is the purpose of this book—"to make you sharp in your thoughts like the sword and decisive enough as a mighty warrior in battlefield."

"To a real warrior, power perceived is the power achieved."

May you all achieve the power of thoughts for the betterment of self and the Society!

The aim of this book is to provide a direction for those pursuing MD/MS/DNB/DGO and passed out candidates searching for next opportunity. It would be a food for thought for all and we are confident that while reading these options you would get a new path to trespass.

All the chapters are written by experts in the respective fields; those who have undergone similar training or are providing training programs.

RECENT TRENDS

Laparoscopy and hysteroscopy are the tools in the armamentarium of the *new age gynecologist* (Fig. 1.2). We all would always want to be well versed with at least basic *endoscopy*. To be frank enough, it would not be a overstatement to say that majority of medical colleges still do not teach hands on endoscopy in the postgraduation (PG) curriculum. Hence, students have to search for this option after their PG course. For the same, we have discussed different courses for learning endoscopy. They are either short duration courses, fellowships, diploma course in India or abroad. We have highlighted the pros and cons of each.

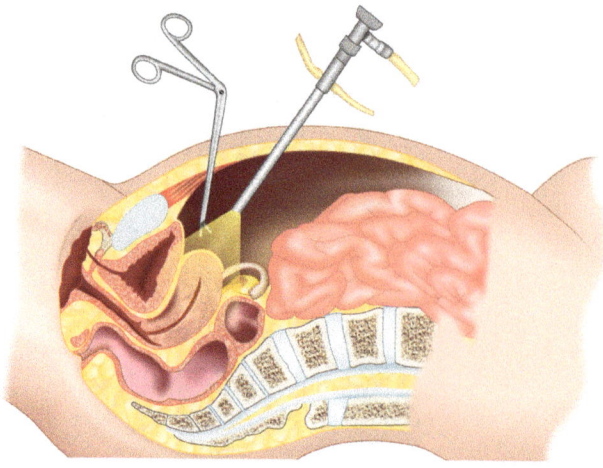

Fig. 1.2: Process of laparoscopy.

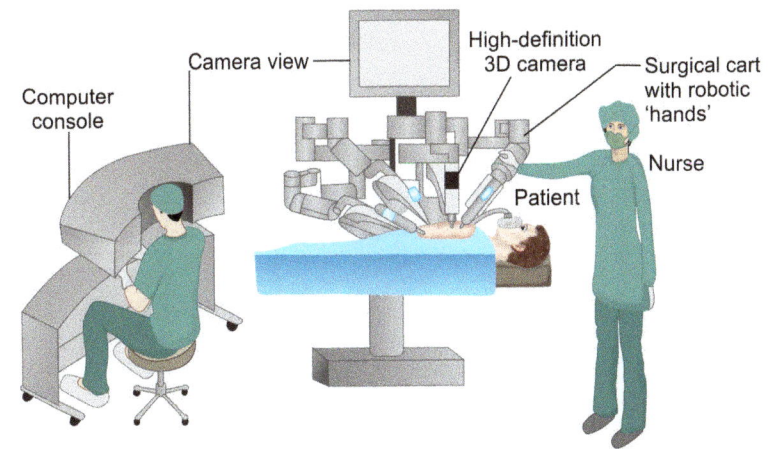

Fig. 1.3: Process of robotic surgery.

Robotic surgery is a little costly option as of today but the ease of surgery, a shorter learning curve and more and more corporate hospitals opting for robotic surgery units have made this field an alluring one (Fig. 1.3). Still there are not much Robotic Centers in India. So many more Robotic surgeons would be needed to meet the *unmet need*.

Gynecologic-oncology is the superspecialty branch which is existent as superspecialty degree course much before other superspecialty branches grew. Tata Memorial Hospital offers MCh courses in Gynecologic Oncology for surgeons as well as gynecologists. Many other colleges are now providing similar courses. One day *colposcopy* courses are also available.

Maternal fetal medicine (MFM) is a specialty branch in US and UK since a long. In India it has grown into fetal medicine and high risk pregnancy as two separate branches. Courses are available at premier institutes. This core obstetrics branch is much needed asset for students. In this era of corporate world and increasing medicolegal cases (MLC), this specialty is much needed.

Reproductive medicine is at the forefront of emerging medico-scientific technology, offering hope to many needy couples, and career opportunities to those with demonstrable skills and knowledge (Fig. 1.4). Much has been known to students as well. But here we have mentioned in detail the fellowship, degree and diploma courses for the same.

Urogynecology is a branch which is definitely growing. Urinary incontinence, prolapse and their repair are best managed by the urogynecologists. Internationally acclaimed surgeons have tried to put light on this field.

The *cosmetic gynecology* course teaches you principles and strategies that tie together with knowledge that you already possess. Regardless of your background, it will give you the foundation to grow in this exciting

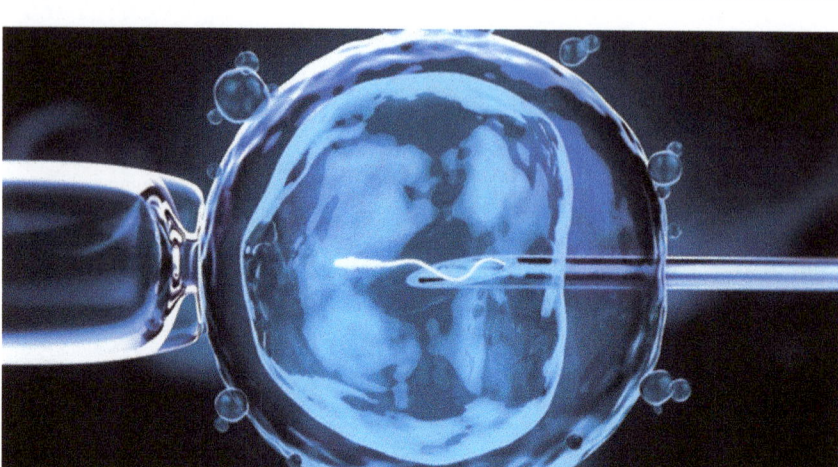

Fig. 1.4: Application of reproductive medicine.

arena. Initially criticized by some, this is a high yielding field with initial high investment.

Some may have missed the chance to settle in the US immediately after their MBBS, might think of appearing for United States Medical Licensing Examination (USMLE) after their MD/MS. The Chapter provides insight for the same.

Maternal and child health (MCH) services form the backbone of health services of any country. Hence, the role of an obstetrics and gynecology (OBGYN) specialist is important for designing and implementing the national programs. Many of our colleagues are already doing great work at the family planning and public health government institutes. Opportunities in this regard are also many in India. Union Public Service Commission (UPSC) and State Service Commissions are conducting the examinations every year which can help you reach the topmost positions. The author for this chapter is herself an OBGYN specialist and giving great services to the local health body. Working in public domain on a larger canvas, more than that of government hospitals, is serving in the capacity of IAS/IPS/IRS officer. The field demands high level dedication while preparing for the examinations, during the difficult training and also during the field posting as officer in-charge. Our own medical colleges have produced the talent which is helping our country to change, prosper and evolve. We are happy to have the IAS/IPS officer writing the chapter for our fraternity.

Sometimes, we think our friends are living a very good, luxurious corporate lifestyle. They too have their share of efforts and problems. But we also do have an opportunity to lead a corporate life and work in the corporate field. Doctors are doing MBA in Hospital Administration and other MBAs to make

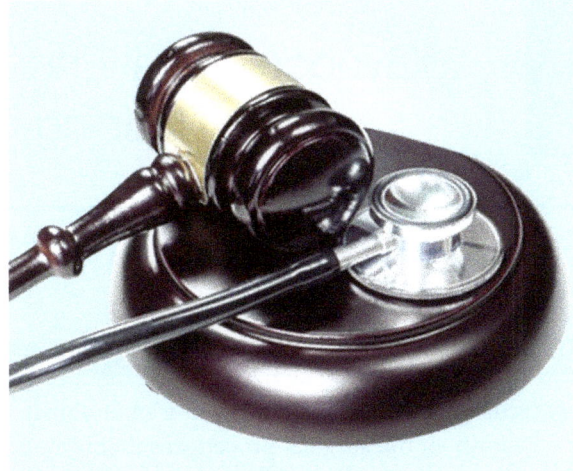

Fig. 1.5: Doctors becoming lawyers.

their talent work in the corporate. Author for this chapter is working in the International arena. Doctors wear apron, the white coat. Radically opposite is the black coat by the lawyers and judges. It is not infrequent for us to take help of our friends from the legal arena in midst of increasing medicolegal hassles, especially in the field of OBGYN (Fig. 1.5). So why not, we as doctors, have lawyers amongst ourselves who can know the intricacies of medical as well as legal fields at the same time (Fig. 1.5). This can help us to protect our colleagues in need. The author being a lawyer and national coordinator for *Medicolegal Committee, FOGSI* has given us tips for the same.

There are endless things and professions which you can practice in your life. Here we have tried to give your insight on few relevant fields.

Hope this fulfills your aspirations and you pave the way for some new beginning!

Every second brings.... a fresh beginning,
Every hour holds....a new promise,
Every night our dreams.... can bring hope, and
Every day is what you choose to make it!

CHAPTER 2

Gynecological Endoscopy Training in India

Sandip Datta Roy

INTRODUCTION

The field of gynecological surgery has evolved tremendously over the last three decades. Majority of the surgical procedures that were being done by traditional laparotomy are now possible with laparoscopic route with all the benefits of minimal invasive surgeries. Lots of progress has been made in hysteroscopic surgeries as well with advent of modern and sophisticated instruments that makes the intrauterine surgeries safe and simple. Slowly and steadily gynecological endoscopic procedures are gaining acceptance both among the gynecological surgeons as well as the patients. Like any other types of surgery, endoscopic gynecological procedures carry the risk of serious complications. Hence, proper understanding of the subject of endoscopy and adequate training is a must before someone ventures into a career of endoscopic surgeries. In this chapter, we will try to give a brief account on the various aspects of training and some of the centers available across the country where candidates can pursue their training depending on their requirements.

In the era of early development of endoscopic surgery, traditional apprenticeship-type programs was common. More recently, formal curricula in endoscopic training have been developed and published. Any formal fellowship training program must incorporate the basic aspect of endoscopy as well as more advanced surgical procedures so that the candidate must understand the subject first and then start doing surgical procedures independently after completion of the training program.

A basic training must provide insight into the physiological changes associated with pneumoperitoneum, superficial and retroperitoneal pelvic anatomy, handling of laparoscopic and hysteroscopic instruments, different access techniques and complications associated with them, principles behind electrosurgery and its application in laparoscopic and hysteroscopic surgeries, tissue retrieval techniques, sterilization of endoscopic instruments, etc. and also how to set up an operating room for endoscopic surgeries.

Once the basic understanding is clear, next stage of training should focus on learning advanced endoscopic procedures by assisting a competent surgeon. Advanced endoscopic training includes the need for advanced endoscopy instrumentation, pelvic endo-trainer exercises for hand-eye coordination, skills development and orientation to different skills, preoperative and postoperative care, operative safety guidelines for different surgeries such as laparoscopic hysterectomy, laparoscopic surgeries for fibroids, severe endometriosis, prolapse repair, pelvic floor defects, benign ovarian tumors, tubal surgeries, etc. and hysteroscopic surgeries for septal resection, submucus fibroid removal, Asherman's syndrome, proximal tubal cannulation, transcervical resection of the endometrium (TCRE), etc. Training under a surgeon with a good volume and variety of cases will allow better exposure and hasten the process of learning advanced endoscopic procedures. As laparoscopy has a longer learning curve, one must spend enough time in pelvic-training sessions on simulators with special emphasis on endosuturing.

DETAILS OF FEW TRAINING CENTERS

Cochin Gynecological Endoscopic Training Center

Under the guidance of Dr PG Paul, this center provides both short-term and long-term training in gynecological endoscopy. Two weeks short-term training is a hands-on program for gynecologist conducted throughout the year. There is also a 1-year fellowship program in gynecological endoscopy. For further details, visit *www.paulshospital.com* or email to *paulhospitaltraining@gmail.com*.

Sunrise Hospitals, Kochi

This center offers basic and advanced laparoscopy training of 12 days. Also there is a fellowship program in advanced gynecological laparoscopy of 6 months duration. The training program is headed by famous laparoscopic surgeon Dr Hafeez Rahman. Details of training programs and the contact details can be obtained from the hospital website *www.sunrisehospitalcochin.com*.

NILES and Aakar IVF Center

Training program is headed by Dr Prakash Trivedi. Address of the center is: 2/3, Gautam Building, Tilak Road, Ghatkopar (East), Mumbai, Maharashtra 400077
Telephone: (022) 67997810/67997809, (022) 25158920
Mobile: 09820052631/09820679777
E-mail: dr.ptrivedi@gmail.com

Akola Endoscopy Center

Training program is headed by Dr Rajesh Modi. Address of the center:
Alsi Plot, Near NCC Office, Akola, Maharashtra-444001
Telephone: 2431290, Mobile: 09823120020
E-mail: rajeshmodi99@hotmail.com

Altius Hospital, Bengaluru

This center provides both basic and advanced gynecological laparoscopic surgeries under the guidance of Dr B Ramesh. It has 1 month, 6 months and 18 months fellowship training programs. Fellowship candidates are selected on the basis of an interview. The contact details can be obtained from the hospital website *www.altiushospital.com.*

Vardhman Trauma and Laparoscopy Center

Training in laparoscopy and hysteroscopic surgeries are provided under the guidance of Dr Nutan Jain. The contact details are:
A-36, South Civil Lines, Mahavir Chowk, Muzaffarnagar, Uttar Pradesh-251001
Telephone: 0131-2623084, 2623085
Fax: 0131-2622737
Mobile: 09837082637.
E-mail: jainnutan@gmail.com,jainnutan@hotmail.com
Website: www.vardhmanhospital.com

Malhotra Nursing and Maternity Home

84, MG Road, Agra, Uttar Pradesh-282010
Telephone: (0562) 2260275/ 309215/2262143,
Fax: (0562) 2265194, Mobile: 09897099331
E-mail: drnarendra@malhotrahospitals.com
Website: www.narendarmalhotra.net

Mayflower Women's Hospital

Training program is headed by Dr Sanjay Patel. Contact details are:
"Mayflower House", 132 Ft., Ring Road-Drive in Road Junction, Opposite Traffic Police Helmet, Near Manavmandir, Memnagar, Ahmedabad-380052
Telephone: 079-27495001/02/03, Mobile: 09824039841
E-mail: contact@mayflowerhospital.com
Website: www.mayflowerhospital.com

Endoworld Hospital Pvt. Ltd.

Training program is headed by Dr Pandit Palaskar. Contact details are as follows:
723, In front of Airport Chikalthana, Aurangabad, Maharashtra-431 007
Telephone: 0240-3058500, *Mobile:* 9372235934, 9422235934, 9422712637
E-mail: dr@panditpalaskar.com; contact@endoworldhospital.com
Website: www.panditpalaskar.com; www.endoworldshospital.com

Nadkarni Medical Training Academy for IVF and Gynaec-Endoscopy

It offers 1 month, 3 months and 6 months fellowship courses. Address of center:
Nadkarni Hospital and Test Tube Baby Center
Char Rasta, N.H. No. 8, Killa Pardi, Valsad, Gujarat-396125
Mobile: 9998743551, 9879507743
E-mail: training@nadkarnihospital.com
Website: www.nadkarniacademy.com

DY Patil University Medical Fellowship Program, Mumbai

Fellowship program is done under the guidance of Dr Neeta Warty. For details, contact: medical.fellowships@dypatil.edu.

Manchanda's Endoscopic Center

This center offers short term training of 1, 2 and 6 weeks for basic endoscopy. Also there are long-term fellowships ranging from 3 months to 2 years.
Mobile: 9810017651
Website: www.gynaeendoscopy.com

Lifeline Hospital

FOGSI recognized center for short training as well as fellowship program in gynecological endoscopy. Contact details are:
Lifeline Hospital, 14th Mile
Melood PO, Adoor, Pathanamthitta District, Kerala
Mobile: 8281264784.
Website: www.lifelinehospitalkerala.com

Ruby Hall Clinic

Dr Sunita Tandulwadkar, Pune, Maharashtra
Mobile: 9822015850
E-mail: sunitart@hotmail.com

Joseph Nursing Home

Dr A Joseph Kurian and Dr Rekha Kurian, Chennai, Tamil Nadu
Telephone: 44-26413254
Mobile: 09840599979
E-mail: drrekhakurian@gmail.com

Sunrise Hospital

Dr Sandesh Kade, Solapur, Maharasthra
Mobile: 9822195070
E-mail: sandesh.kade@gmail.com

Pragnesh J Shah

Jyoti Maternity Hospital and Minimum
Invasive Surgery Center, Ocean Park,
Satellite Road, Ahmedabad, Gujarat-380015
Telephone: 91-79-26731759/26766491
Mobile: 9824050916/9824450916
Fax: 91-79-26766491
Email: pragnesh.j.shah@gmail.com; pragnesh@laparoscopyexpert.com
Website: www.laparoscopyexpert.com

Ratna Kaul

Kaul Hospital and Research Center
Naya Bazar, Gwalior, Madhya Pradesh-474009
Mobile: 9425109900/982625331
E-mail: dockaulhospital@yahoo.in

Malvika Sabharwal

Jeewan Mala Hospital
New Rohtak Road, New Delhi 110005
Telephone: 011-9212204348
Mobile: 9810116293
E-mail: ms@jeewanmalahospital.com

KV Argade

Maher Gynecology, Endoscopy and Infertility Center,
Maternity and Gynecology Nursing Home, 8th Lane
Rajarampuri, Kolhapur, Maharasthra-416008
Telephone: (0231)-2521371/2521740/2528150
Mobile: 9822044895/9423856895
E-mail: kvargade@sancharnet.in

KK Gopinathan

Center for Infertility Management and Assisted Reproduction
Edappal Hospitals Pvt. Ltd., Edappal, Kerala-679576
Telephone: 0494-2680755/0494-2681788, 0494-2680798/0494-2680448
Mobile: 9846102429/9847013900
E-mail: cimar@eth.net; cimarindia@sancharnet.in

Manju Jilla

Dr Jilla Hospital
84, Motiwala Nagar, Centra Naka Road, Aurangabad, Maharashtra-431005
Mobile: 9822030485
Telephone: (0240) 2337245, 2337346
Fax: (0240) 2331036, 2335200.
E-mail: manju.jilla@rediffmail.com

Parul Kotdawala

Kotdawala Women's Clinic
53/1, Brahmin Mitra Mandal Society, Opp. Jalaram Temple, Near Old Sharda Mandir Railway Crossing, Ellisbridge, Ahmedabad, Gujarat-380006
Telephone: (079) 26575813, 26580322
Fax No.: (079) 26576107
Mobile: 9426725267
E-mail: kotdawala@dataone.in, kotdawala@yahoo.com

S Krishnakumar

JK Women Hospital
Maitri Raghukul, Shaheed Bhagat Singh Road, Opp. Saraswat Bank Dombivli (E), Maharashtra-421 201
Telephone: 0251-2444421/2444431, 0251-2444441/2444405
Mobile: 7045947047
E-mail: jkwomenhospital@gmail.com

Y Savitha Devi

Swapna Health Care
6-3-1111/19, Nishath Bagh, Begumpet, Hyderabad, Telangana-500016
Telephone: 040-2340 2417/2340-5019, 2341 2523
Mobile: 96180 61277
Fax: 91-040-2340 0439
E-mail: swapnahealthcare@gmail.com
Website: www.swapnahealthcare.com

K Jayakrishnan

Director/Chief Medical Officer
KJK Hospital, Shawallace Lane, Nalanchira
Thiruvananthapuram, Kerala-695015
Telephone: 0471-2544080, 0471-2544705/2544706
E-mail: kjkhospital@rediffmail.com, kjkhospital@gmail.com
Website: www.kjkhospital.com

Vineet Mishra

Institute of Kidney Disease and Research Center
BJ Medical College and Civil Hospital Campus
Ahmedabad, Gujarat-380016
Telephone: 079-27455699, 079-2268000
Mobile: 09426078333
E-mail: vvmishra@yahoo.com

Mehul Sukhadiya

Sumiran Women's Hospital
46-B-2, Swastik Society, Near Vodafone House
Stadium Five Road, Stadium Commerce Six Road
Navrangpura, Ahmedabad, Gujarat-380009
Telephone: 079-26464697
Mobile: 7622000425/421
E-mail: mehulsukhadiya@yahoo.com, radhehospital119@gmail.com

Vasundhara Kamineni

Department of Gynecology and Obstetrics
Kamineni Hospital Ltd.
Ring Road, LB Nagar, Hyderabad, Andhra Pradesh-500068
Telephone: 040-24022272 to 76/39879999/24022222
Fax: 040-24022277
E-mail: kamineni@kamineni.org
Website: www.kaminenihospitals.com

Chaitanya Shembekar

21, Ashirwad, Ramkrishna Nagar, Ajni Square
Khamla Road, Nagpur, Maharashtra-440015
Telephone: 0712-2221807/0712-2454687
Mobile: 0-9822572744
E-mail: chaitanyashembekar@yahoo.com

Meenu Agarwal

Morpheus Bliss Fertility Center, A-7/8, Siddharth Court, 1st Floor
Dhole Patil Road, Pune, Maharashtra-411001
Telephone: 020-41265050
Mobile: 09822036970
E-mail: drmjainagarwal@hotmail.com
Website: www.morpheus_art.com

Anupama Sethi Arora

Saxena Multispeciality Hospital Pvt. Ltd.
112-113, TP Scheme, Delhi Road, Sonepat, Haryaya-131001
Telephone: 0130-2232211, 2218811
Mobile: 0-9315145824, 9996004919, 9355584919
E-mail: anupama.ivf@gmail.com, amar_hospital@hotmail.com

Asha Baxi

Disha Fertility and Surgical Center
E-30, Saket Nagar (Extn.), Indore, Madhya Pradesh-452001
Telephone: 0731-2565768, 2565755
Mobile: 0-9826056576
E-mail: aabaxi@gmail.com

Anita Singh

Chief Consultant
Jyoti Punj Hospital, Boring Road, Patna, Bihar-800001
Telephone: 0612-2540752, 3259563, 0612-2221341
Mobile: 0-9334111925
E-mail: sanita51@sify.com

Tejas Dave

Pooja Hospital
33, Prankunj Society, Pushpkunj, Kankaria, Ahmedabad, Gujarat-390028
Telephone: 079-25332776/25332176
Mobile: 09825063132
E-mail: jignatejasdave@yahoo.com

Minaxi Patel

Global Baroda Hospital
Near Nalani House, Manjalpur, Vadodara, Gujarat-390001
Telephone: 0265-3300400/0265-3938200
Mobile: 9825112478
E-mail: mbpgbh@gmail.com, care@globalbarodahospital.com

Manoj Chellani

Aayush Hospital and Maternity Home
C-9, Ashok Ratan VIP Estate, Vidhan Sabha Road, Shankar Nagar
Khamardih, Raipur, Chhattisgarh-492001
Mobile: 09826611688
E-mail: drmanoj22@gmail.com

Chetna Jain

Preksha Hospital
Plot No. 4, Main Pal Road, Jodhpur, Rajasthan
Mobile: 09829009726/09414126802
E-mail: jainpravin4@gmail.com

Dinesh Kansal/Alka Sinha

Dr BL Kapur Memorial Hospital
Pusa Road, New Delhi-110005
Telephone: 011-30403040
Mobile (Dr. Dinesh Kansal): 09810884822
Mobile (Dr Alka Sinha): 09312071293
E-mail: info@blkhospital.com

Archana Baser

Akash Hospital and Diagnostic Center
Bicholi, Mardana, Main Road, Opposite Agrawal Public School
Indore, Madhya Pradesh-452001
Telephone: 0731-2847039, 2847040
Mobile: 8305464080/7869914080/9826064080
E-mail: archanabaser@gmail.com, akashhosp@gmail.com

D Rama Krishna Hanuman

Sankar Laparoscopy and Infertility Center
Sankar Nursing Home, Prakasam District, Chirala, Andhra Pradesh-523155
Mobile: 09848152056/09441282086
E-mail: nitahans@yahoo.com

L Fahmida Banu

Fehmi Care Hospital
8-3-229/37 Tahir Villa, Yousuf Ganda Checkpost
Hyderabad, Telangana-500045
Mobile: 09246544465
E-mail: dr_lfahmida@yahoo.com

Vaishali Tandon

Dr Kamlesh Tandon Hospital and Test Tube Baby Center
4/48 Lajpat Kunj, Bag Farzana
Agra, Uttar Pradesh-282002
Telephone: 0562-2521569, 2525369
Mobile: 09837053990
E-mail: drkamleshtandonhospital@yahoo.com

Bimal M John

Credence Hospital Pvt. Ltd.
Near Ulloor Bridge, Ulloor, Medical College P.O.
Thiruvananthapuram, Kerala-695011
Mobile: 9895375279
E-mail: bimaljohn@gmail.com

Vidya Bhat

Radhakrishna Multispeciality Hospital and IVF Center
3-4 Sunrise Tower, JP Road
Girinagar, Bengaluru, Karnataka-560085
Telephone: 26422977/988
Telefax: 080-26720222
Mobile: 098820106354
E-mail: vidyabhat68@gmail.com

Divyesh Shukla

Isha Hospital
Behind Atlantis, Opposite Vadodara Central
Sarabhai Campus, Sarabhai Main Road
Vadodara, Gujarat-390007
Telephone: 0265-2314011/2314022
Mobile: 98250 61950
E-mail: info@ishahospital.com

Devang Kanuga/Manish Shah

Grace Endoscopy Center
Women's Institute of Infertility and Gynecology Endoscopic
Surgery (WINGS), 2, Sumangalam Society; Opposite Drive-in Cinema
Bodakdev, Ahmedabad, Gujarat-380054
Mobile: 98250 50565, 9375050565

Sanjay Makwana and Renu Makwana

Vasundhara Hospital and Fertility Research Center
11/11, Nandanwan, Near Chopasani Housing
Board Office
Jodhpur, Rajasthan 342001
Telephone: 0291-2710401/402/403
Mobile: 9829026402
E-mail: vhfrc.jodhpur@gmail.com, vasundharafertility@yahoo.com
Website: www.vasundharafertility.com

Mukesh Agrawal

Aarush IVF and Endoscopy Center
1st Floor, Prathamesh Harmony, Gautam Buddha Lane, Opp. Orlem Church
Off Marve Road, Malad (W)
Mumbai, Maharashtra-400064
Telephone: 022-2806 0051/52/53
E-mail: info@aarushivf.com
Website: www.aarushivf.com

Sandeep Mane

The Origin International Fertility Center
Opp. Hiranandani Meadows, Pokhran Road No. 2
Thane (W), Maharashtra-400610
Telephone: 022-21712333/45/40
E-mail: training@theoriginfertility.com

S Pappachan

Managing Director
Lifeline Super Speciality Hospital
4th Mile, Melood, P.O., Pathanamthitta
District: Adoor, Kerala 691523
Telephone: 04734-223377, 221388, 226520, 223488, 325867
Mobile: 9447091144
E-mail: info@lifelinehospitalkerala.com

Meena Naik

Dr Meena Naik Clinic and Training Center
B-198, Street 7, Smriti Nagar, Bhilai, Chhattisgarh-490020
Mobile: 8878226671
E-mail: m.naik1971@yahoo.com

Renu Singh

Gahlaut Health Care Pvt. Ltd.
C-13, New Azad Nagar (Behind Petrol Pump)
Kalyanpur, Kanpur, Uttar Pradesh
Telephone: 0512-2570373, 9839308777
E-mail: renusingh3003@gmail.com
Website: www.gahlauthealthcare.com

Bharati Dhorepatil

"Ssmile" IVF Test Tube Baby Center and
Reproductive Medicine Unit
Shree Hospital, Siddharth Mansion, Nagar Road
Pune, Maharashtra-411006
Telephone: 020 26681127/26684520
Mobile: 9822043112
E-mail: info@shreehospital.com

Bina Goel

Director
Kamla Nagar Hospital
Pal Link Road
Jodhpur, Rajasthan 342 008
Telephone: 0291-2753466, 2753477
Mobile: 9414196855
E-mail: kamlanagarhospital@gmail.com

Pravin Jain

Preksha Hospital and Chetna IVF Research Center
4, Main Pal Road
Jodhpur, Rajasthan-342008
Telephone: 0291–2787000, 2787001
Mobile: 9414126802
E-mail: prekshahospital@gmail.com, jainpravin@gmail.

Anju Soni

Soni Hospital
38, Kanota Bagh, Jawahar Lal Nehru Marg
Jaipur, Rajasthan-302004
Telephone: 0141-5163700
E-mail: sonihospital@sonihospitals.com

Sunil Shah

Yashshree Nursing Home
Ashok Nagar, Behind State Bank of India
Bhigwan Road, Baramati, Maharashtra, Pune-413102
Telephone: 02112-224155/222607
Mobile: 9822979426
E-mail: drsunilshah09@gmail.com

Vaman Ghodake

Dr vaman's Institute for Advanced Laparoscopic Surgeries Research and Training Centers
Central Plaza, 1st Floor, Near Shirgaonkar Blood Bank
Civil Hospital Chowk, Sangli, Maharashtra-416216
Telephone: 0233-2622092/2622290
Mobile: 9970542044/9404290290
E-mail: drvamanghodake@rediffmail.com

Deepak Desh

Rajdeep Fertility Research Center
"Rajdeep Niwas", Near Central Academy School
Saraswati Colony
Baran Road, Kota, Rajasthan-324001
Telephone: 0744-2331122
Mobile: 9829038062

Victo A Wotsa

Director
Nikos Hospital and Research Center
Midland, Dimapur, Nagaland 797112
Telephone: 03862-232032/248285/9436004198
Mobile: 9436004198
E-mail: victo_00@yahoo.com

Mala Raj

Managing Director
Firm Hospitals, R-Block, 65
Annanagar, Chennai, Tamil Nadu-600040
Telephone: 044-26262666 (4 lines)
Mobile: 08056225577
E-mail: drmalaraj@firmhospitals.com

Shivani Sachdev Gour

SCI International Hospital
M-4, Greater Kailash-1, New Delhi-110048
Telephone: 011-41041131/29242429
E-mail: info@scihospital.com

Rekha Bhandari

Bhandari Hospital and Research Center
138-A, Vasundhara Colony, Gopalpura Bypass,
Tonk Road, Jaipur, Rajasthan-302018
Telephone: 0141-2703851/52
Mobile: 9829110044
E-mail: contact@bhandarihospital.net

Neeta Kanwar

Kanwar Nursing Home
TV Tower Road
Shankar Nagar, Raipur, Chhattisgarh-492007
Mobile: 7773013084
E-mail: kanwarnursinghome@yahoo.com

Deepak Goenka

Institute of Human Reproduction (IHR)
Bharalumukh, Guwahati, Assam-781009
Telephone: 0361-2482619/621, 09864103333
E-mail: office@ihrindia.com

Anshu Jindal

Jindal Hospital and Nursing Home
Eves Crossing, Hapur Road, Meerut-250001, Uttar Pradesh
Telephone: 0121-4000444/2642839/2642599
Mobile: 8006666004
E-mail: jindalhospital@gmail.com/jindalart@gmail.com

Satya Narayan Sharma

Dishari Health Point Pvt Ltd.
19, GB Road, PO Mokdumpur
Malda, West Bengal-732103
Mobile: 9434057580
E-mail: dishari_hp@yahoo.co.in

Aruna Tantia

ILS Hospitals
DD- 6, Salt Lake City, Kolkata, West Bengal-700064
Mobile: 9830400445
E-mail: arunatantia@gmail.com

Alka Jain

Sehgal Neo Hospital
B-362, 363, 364, Meera Bagh, Outer Ring Road, New Delhi-110063
Telephone: 011-45565656
Mobile: 9810062631
E-mail: alkagoeljain@yahoo.com

Pramod Kumar Sharma

Pratiksha Hospital
Borbari, Hengrabari, VIP Road, Guwahati, Assam-781036
Telephone: 0361-7101600
E-mail: contact@pratikshahospital.in

Jyoti Malik

JJ Institute of Medical Science Pvt Ltd.
MIE, Part- B, Bahadurgarh, Haryana 174507
Mobile: 7056100100/108/103
E-mail: ms@jjmedicalinstitute.com

Jyoti Mishra

Jaypee Healthcare Ltd
Wish Town, Sector 128,
Noida, Uttar Pradesh-201304
Telephone: 0120-4122222
Mobile: 09958989170
E-mail: drjyotimishra1@gmail.com

Manjula Anagani

Suyosha Health Care Pvt. Ltd.
Plot No. 7, Survey No-64
Patrika Nagar, Madhapur, Hyderabad, Telangana-500081
Mobile: 9848030121
E-mail: drradheeobg@yahoo.com, manjuanagani@yahoo.com

Neena Singh/Dr Madhu Goel

Fortis La Femme
S-549, Greater Kailash II, New Delhi 110048
Telephone: 011-40579400
Mobile: 9871108802
E-mail: contactus.flf@fortishealthcare.com

Kiran S Coelho

Lilavati Hospital and Research Center
A-791, Bandra Reclamation, Bandra (W), Mumbai, Maharashtra-400050
E-mail: kirancoelho@icloud.com

Nisha Jain Gupta

Saroj Super Speciality Hospital
Plot No. 2, Institutional Area Sec-14
Madhuban Chowk, Rohini, Delhi-110085
Mobile: 9810085300/9818656636
E-mail: chawlakiran00@gmail.com, k.chawla@sarojhospital.com
info@sarojhospital.com

Praful Doshi

Me and Mummy Hospital
Jalnidhi Complex, Opp. Bahumali,
Nanpura, Surat, Gujarat-395001
Telephone: 0261-2471111/2472222/9825134253
E-mail: prafuldoshi57@gmail.com, drakp28@gmail.com

Alka Sen

Sen Maternity and Eye Hospital Pvt. Ltd.
44, Gazanan Nagar Kothi, Meena Bazar, Shahganj
Agra, Uttar Pradesh-282010
Mobile: 9359906674
E-mail: dralkasenagra@gmail.com

Nitin Lal

Manan Institute for Fertility Management and Test Tube Baby Center Pvt. Ltd.
Manan Hospital, 25 New Jagnath Main Road
Near Dr. Koshiya Hospital, Rajkot, Gujarat-360001
Telephone: 0281-2480510
E-mail: lalmanan@yahoo.in, mananivf@gmail.com
drsudhirshah@gmail.com

Himanshu Roy

Shivam Hospital and Research Institute Pvt. Ltd.
Vidhyapuri, Kankarbagh, Patna, Bihar-800020
Telephone: 0612-2358713/8002005005
E-mail: himanshuroy@hotmail.com

Sushila Saini

Jaipur Doorbeen Hospital
8, Devi Nagar Mode
NS Road, Jaipur, Rajasthan-302019
Mobile: 9001795896
E-mail: sainisush@yahoo.com

Shrikant Ohri

New Life Center for Advance Laparoscopy
New Life Hospital, 70, Gandhi Nagar
Sigra, Varanasi, Uttar Pradesh-221010
Telephone: 0542-2221293, 2220036
Mobile: 8932055555
E-mail: info@newlife.com, shrikant_391@hotmail.com

CP Dadhich

Eternal Hospital
Jaipur Chainpura, Near Jawahar Circle
Jaipur, Rajasthan-302017
Mobile: 9829217530
E-mail: cpdadhich_dr@yahoo.com

L Priya

Aakash Hospital and Aaditya Fertility Center
393/1, TH Road, Thiruvottiyur, Chennai, Tamil Nadu-600019
Mobile: 9500027502
E-mail: aadityafertility@gmail.com

Rooma Sinha

Apollo Hospital
Jubilee Hills, Hyderabad, Telangana-96
Mobile: 9849008180
E-mail: drroomasinha@hotmail.com

B Sandhya Rani

Laxmi Narasimha Hospital
2-2-316, Naim Nagar, Krishanpura, Hanamkonda
Warangal-506001, Telengana
Mobile: 9550563366
E-mail: sandhyarani133@gmail.com

Vijay Nahata

Mahatma Gandhi Hospital and Medical College
Sitapura, Jaipur, Rajasthan-302022
Mobile: 9864027516
E-mail: vsnahata@gmail.com

CONCLUSION

Apart from these training centers, there are many other centers and individual doctors providing short term as well as fellowship training programs in minimally invasive gynecological endoscopic surgeries. Due to space constraints, it is not possible to include all of them in this chapter. The details of such training centers can be found in FOGSI (Federation of Obstetric and Gynaecological Societies of India) and IAGE (Indian Association of Gynaecological Endoscopists) websites.

Just taking training in endoscopic surgeries may not be the only factor for a successful career in gynecological endoscopy. A trained person must ensure availability of all necessary instruments and preferably work in a place with good volume of cases immediately after completion of the training. Working with a senior and established surgeon for sometimes is also a good idea. Complications can happen more frequently in the early stages of independent practice and one should not hesitate to take help from senior and experienced surgeons to manage them. Doing more of simple cases initially can boost the confidence and gradually one can start performing more complicated cases with greater degree of safety.

CHAPTER 3

Minimal Invasive Surgery (International)

K Subash Mallya

LIST OF LAPAROSCOPIC TRAINING CENTERS OUTSIDE INDIA

Minimally invasive surgical techniques are progressively replacing conventional open techniques. Laparoscopy, in both its conventional form and its recent modalities has been found to be associated with better cosmetic results, shorter hospitalization, less postoperative pain and faster recovery. The introduction of a certification program in minimal invasive surgery (MIS) is expected to improve surgical performance, patient's safety and outcome. A big number of gynecologists practicing MIS today did not follow a proper lab and or animal training prior to operate on humans. Today a young gynecologist interested in practicing laparoscopy and or hysteroscopy should first have excellent theoretical knowledge, training in simulators, animal models, and exercise in dry and wet lab. Due to these limitations, consultants in medical education agree that part of the training has to take place outside the operating room, and various animal and artificial models have been proposed. Animal models seem ideal because they imitate the human clinical scenario in a very realistic manner. The gaining of surgical competence is a continuous learning process, demanding one-to-one learning with a highly skilled surgeon.

To counteract the diversity in strategies and regulations for training in gynecological laparoscopy, there is an urgent need to use a validated system for credentialing an individual's skills. Many academies in collaboration with the European Society of Gynaecological Endoscopy (ESGE) and European Board and College of Obstetrics and Gynaecology (EBCOG) are in the final phase of defining a global program of certification for gynecological laparoscopic surgery. The certification of an individual surgeon is based on *four* criteria, namely practical laparoscopic technical skills, theoretical skills, surgical experience and continuous medical education (CME) accreditation in laparoscopic surgical educational programs. Adopting new instruments and techniques has been the result of the continuous technological advancements while the importance of ergonomics, training and testing only recently gained interest and importance. The following list is just to give an idea of the training centers outside India.

CICE—FRANCE

It consists of a training program developed by the European Academy of Gynaecological Surgery (EAGS) and the ESGE. This course offers candidates not only the theoretical and practical training courses usually given in Clermont-Ferrand, but also the opportunity of obtaining the new European certification in gynecological endoscopy at the end of these 2 weeks of training. This institute is very famous among gynecologists looking for advanced training in laparoscopy.

Website: http://www.cice.fr/index.php/en/contact

THE EUROPEAN ACADEMY OF GYNAECOLOGICAL SURGERY

The academy organizes courses on laparoscopy and hysteroscopy on a regular basis. These courses are designed to be hands-on, with exposure to the latest instruments and minimal invasive techniques. Practical exercises are combined with lectures by experts and, depending on the course, live surgery sessions.

The academy has, in collaboration with the ESGE, developed two certification programs: (1) the GESEA PROGRAMME and the (2) DIGESTT PROGRAMME. The GESEA program offers a pathway to acquire the necessary knowledge and practical skills to become a minimal invasive gynecological surgeon, while the DIGESTT program combines ultrasound imaging with minimal invasive techniques.

Training centers are located at Austria, Belgium, France, Italy, and Portugal.

Website: https://europeanacademy.org/

BSGE—BRITISH SOCIETY FOR GYNAECOLOGICAL ENDOSCOPY

The BSGE exists to improve standards, promote training and encourage the exchange of information in minimal access surgery techniques for women with gynecological problems. The academy organizes courses on laparoscopy and hysteroscopy on a regular basis. These courses are designed to be hands-on, with exposure to the latest instruments and minimal invasive techniques. Practical exercises are combined with lectures by experts and, depending on the course and live surgery sessions.

Website: https://www.bsge.org.uk/contact/

LAPAROSCOPIC INSTITUTE FOR GYNECOLOGY AND ONCOLOGY, USA

Devoted to training of gynecologic general and oncologic surgeons in minimally invasive laparoscopic procedures, Laparoscopic Institute for

Gynecology and Oncology (LIGO) is the only training institute of its kind. Through an intensive hands-on course, LIGO has trained over 2,400 gynecologic surgeons from around the world.

Website: https://ligocourses.com/contact-us/

DUNDEE INSTITUTE FOR HEALTHCARE SIMULATION, UK

The center acts as a focus for multidisciplinary teaching and faculties are drawn from practicing clinicians and other experts who ensure the high quality and relevance of the courses. The training covers predominantly, but not exclusively, endoscopic skills at three levels: (1) basic, (2) advanced and (3) procedure related.

Website: https://cuschieri.dundee.ac.uk/contact-us.

AECS—DUBAI

This institute is committed to provide high quality medical training courses with CME credit hours approved by Dubai Health Authority DHA to doctors, gynecologists, obstetricians, sonographers. Their certificate programs are endorsed by world's leading universities and societies during this course students will learn about past, present, and future of endoscopic gynecological surgery, instruments handling, abdominal entry, suturing and knot-tying techniques. They will also learn hand-eye-coordination and operative hysteroscopy. This gynecological endoscopy course is endorsed by Kiel School of Gynecological Endoscopy, Germany—Society of Laparoscopy Surgeon (SLS), USA—The International Society of Gynecological Endoscopy (ISGE), Europe—Universitatsklinikum Schleswig-Holsten (UKSH), Germany.

Website: https://www.aecsmed.com/contact-us

KIEL SCHOOL OF ENDOSCOPY, GERMANY

The Kiel School of Gynaecological Endoscopy sees itself as a modern-style training school. This applies to its very active educational function as well as its well-equipped training school and operating room. The Kiel School is a certified training center of the German Society of Gynaecological Endoscopy (AGE). Since the 1970s the Kiel Department of Obstetrics and Gynaecology has been a pioneer in the field of endoscopy. This is by far the most popular training centers for Indians.

E-mail: kiel.school@uksh.de
Website: https://www.kiel-school.de/kiel_school/en/Contact.html

INTERNATIONAL SOCIETY FOR GYNECOLOGIC ENDOSCOPY—FELLOWSHIPS

The International Society for Gynecologic Endoscopy (ISGE) was formed in 1989 by a group committed endoscopists from Europe and North America, who were soon joined by others from all over the world. This program will be structured so that the accreditation will be of academic and legal value in the specific country where the specific member applying for ISGE accreditation.

To achieve this goal the ISGE Task Force for the Accreditation of Gynecological Endoscopy (TFAGE), under the guidance of the ISGE President Professor Bruno van Herendael, has called on a world renowned specialist in accreditation Professor Walter Costantini of Milan University in Italy. They have together elaborated the ISGE accreditation program.

Website: https://www.isge.org/isge-contact-information

APAGE—TAIWAN

The Asia-Pacific Association for Gynecologic Endoscopy and Minimally Invasive Therapy (APAGE) represents over 15 associations in the gynecologic field worldwide. The main training center is located at Chang Gung Memorial Hospital in Linkou, Taiwan.

Short-time Fellowship

Doctors whom would like to observe advanced laparoscopic and hysteroscopic surgery can apply for the short-term program which is 1–3 months.
Observation only (Hands-off).

Clinical Fellowship

Doctors whom are interested in hands-on surgical training can apply for the long-term program which is designed for experienced doctors whom interested in gynecological oncology and minimal invasive surgery. The period of attachment is limited to 1–2 years.
- Hands-on practice (depends on mentors' evaluation)
- Case study research
- Surgical video editing
- Individual mentoring.

Certification

The trainees whom completed the short-term fellowship program will obtain certificate from the APAGE

Website: http://www.apagemit.com/page/contact/index.aspx

MINIMAL ACCESS SURGICAL TRAINING, UK

The minimal access surgical training (MAST) center is running 2-day courses in hysteroscopy and laparoscopy, which is primarily intended for *SHOs and Specialist Registrars in Gynecology.*

The training and accreditation needs for the hysteroscopy course are in conjunction with the Royal College of Obstetricians and Gynaecologists (RCOG) levels of surgical competencies required. The main aim for the hysteroscopy course is to achieve advanced level competency (RCOG special skills module), which equates to being able to perform endometrial ablation using resection/rollerball technique.

Website: http://mymds.bham.ac.uk/mast/hyst.asp

ITALIAN SCHOOL OF ENDOSCOPY

Italian School of Endoscopy (ISE) is a medical education project born from the ideas and experiences of young gynecologists and surgeons with proven skills in the field of minimally invasive gynecological surgery. ISE offers to its members the opportunity to spend a training period abroad in hospitals, universities, and private clinics who stand out in the field of minimally invasive gynecological surgery.

This training is intended as a fellowship or observership (depending on the country of destination), and takes place in periods ranging from 1 month to 3 months.

Available locations:
- Italy
- Europe (Germany, UK, Romania, Slovenia)
- USA (Wisconsin, Virginia, Florida, Georgia, Pennsylvania)
- Brazil.

At the end of the training period it will be released a certificate indicating the period, the location, and the achievements of the training program.

ISE courses in Laparoscopy:
- Laparoscopy: Level 1
- Laparoscopy: Level 2
- Laparoscopy: Level 3
- Laparoscopy: Level 4

Website: http://www.ise.surgery/en/contacts/

MINIMAL ACCESS SURGERY DIPLOMA (OLDENBURG, GERMANY)

It is a German diploma in basic and advanced laparoscopic surgery. A comprehensive training program in basic and advanced laparoscopy with training at Oldenburg, Germany.
- Hands-on live surgery
- In basic endoscopic surgery for 1 day
- Advanced gynecological endoscopic surgeries for 4 days
- Minimal invasive/hysteroscopy surgeries for 1 day

Diploma endorsed by:
- University Hospital for Gynecology, Carl von Ossietzky University, Oldenburg
- European Society for Gynecological Endoscopy (ESGE)
- German academy of Obstetrics and Gynecology (DGGG)
- German Association of Gynecological Endoscopy (AGE)

E-mail: zimtconferences@gmail.com
Website: http://www.zimtdubai.com/masdiploma/

The influence of such an educational and credentialing path could improve the safety and offer financial benefits to the hospitals, physicians, and healthcare authorities. Moreover the medicolegal consequences can be important when a significant amount of surgeons possess the different diplomas. As the programs are becoming universally accessible, recognized as the best scientific standard, included in the CME and professional development (CPD), I do expect that a significant number of surgeons will soon accomplish the diploma path. Please note this list is not exhaustive and only includes some of the most common and popular centers.

SUMMARY

1. CICE—France
   http://www.cice.fr/index.php/en/contact
2. The European Academy of Gynaecological Surgery
   https://europeanacademy.org/
3. BSGE—British Society for Gynaecological Endoscopy
   https://www.bsge.org.uk/contact/
4. Institute for Gynecology and Oncology (LIGO), USA
   https://ligocourses.com/contact-us/
5. Dundee Institute for Healthcare Simulation, UK
   https://cuschieri.dundee.ac.uk/contact-us.
6. AECS, Dubai
   https://www.aecsmed.com/contact-us
7. Kiel School of Endoscopy
   https://www.kiel-school.de/kiel_school/en/Contact.html
8. ISGE Fellowships
   https://www.isge.org/isge-contact-information
9. APAGE, Taiwan
   http://www.apagemit.com/page/contact/index.aspx
10. MAST, UK
    http://mymds.bham.ac.uk/mast/hyst.asp
11. Italian School of Endoscopy
    http://www.ise.surgery/en/contacts/
12. MAS Diploma, Oldenburg, Germany
    E-mail: zimtconferences@gmail.com, http://www.zimtdubai.com/masdiploma/

CHAPTER 4

Robotic Surgery: Next Frontier in Minimal Invasive Surgery

Rajendra P Shitole

OVERVIEW

Minimally invasive surgical procedures avoid open invasive surgery in favor of closed or local surgery with less trauma. These procedures can often be done vaginally or involve use of laparoscopic instruments. Laparoscopy allows observation of the surgical field through an endoscope or similar device, and is carried out through small incisions in the skin to allow access into the pelvis or abdomen. This may result in shorter hospital stays, or allow outpatient treatment.

The da Vinci® system is a robotic operating system (Fig. 4.1), approved by the US Food and Drug Administration (FDA) for gynecologic surgery in 2005, is one of the newest technologies available for the treatment of gynecologic problems including hysterectomy and ovarian surgery for cancer and other conditions such as pelvic organ prolapse.

For most patients, robotic surgery can offer numerous potential benefits over traditional approaches to vaginal, laparoscopic or open abdominal hysterectomy, particularly when performing more challenging procedures

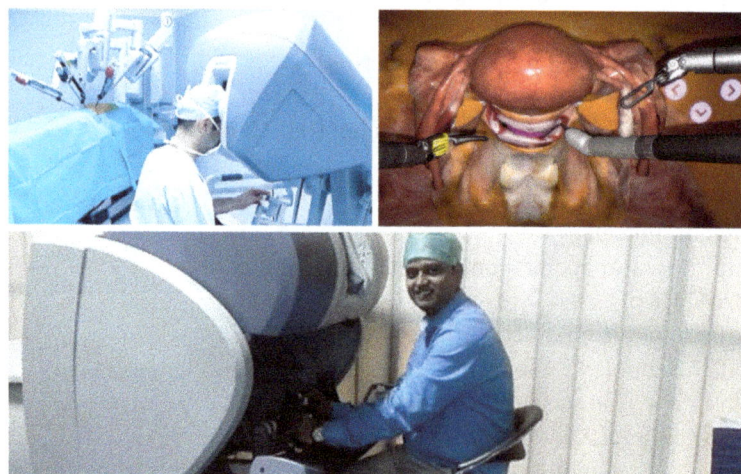

Fig. 4.1: Robotic operating system

like radical hysterectomy for gynecologic cancer or sacrocolpopexy for pelvic organ prolapse. Potential benefits include:
- Significantly less pain
- Less blood loss
- Fewer complications
- Less scarring
- A shorter hospital stay
- A faster return to normal daily activities

It enables gynecologists to offer an effective minimally invasive approach for benign gynecologic conditions requiring surgery. Compared to conventional laparoscopic surgery, robotic assistance minimizes conversions as well as the need for total abdominal hysterectomy. The excellent visualization (3D HD vision), dexterity (EndoWrist instrumentation) and control (intuitive motion) provide surgeons with a surgical option to approach pathology minimally invasively, safely, reproducibly and even in high risk patients with adhesive disease, obesity.

In gynecology robotic surgery has many applications:
1. Benign hysterectomies (fibroids, AUB)
2. Surgeries for prolapse, SUI (sacrocolpopexy, hysteropexy, burch colposuspension)
3. Endometriosis
4. Gynecological oncology

Success in adoption of a surgical modality is highly dependent of the learning curve associated with acquisition of the necessary skills to comfortably and efficiently perform it. For the surgeon, robotic surgery overcomes some problems of conventional laparoscopic surgery. Muscular efforts are minimized because improved ergonomics when sitting at a console separate from the patient. Furthermore, combination of improved imaging and instrument control could allow for a faster surgical learning curve compared with conventional laparoscopy, which includes two-dimensional imaging and counterintuitive hand movements. However, even if the use of robot-assisted technology is believed to shorten the learning curve of complex minimally invasive procedures, the number of cases required for proficiency in robotic-assisted gynecological surgery is not clear.

Surgeons should be skilled at abdominal and laparoscopic approaches for a specific procedure before undertaking robotic approaches.

OPTIONS AVAILABLE FOR TRAINING IN ROBOTIC GYNECOLOGY

Institutional

- Institutions where robotic systems have been purchased and if you are working there, institute can send you or you can go for training through intuitive surgical at designated centers.

- If you are working in other institute where robotic system is not available, but you are interested in learning robotic then you can apply to that institution for getting access to console and if institute is ready for same then you can apply for training through that institute with the help of da Vinci® representative.

It is a phasic training which includes online modules, training at institute level, hands on training on porcine (animal) lab at designated centers, hands on training at parent institute under mentor guidance, advanced hands on training cadavers in sequential manner. Cost of training is approximately *3,000 USD*. After completing training you will be designated as a console surgeon. You can check out details at *davincisurgerycommunity.com*.

Da Vinci® Training Passport Technology Training Pathway: Surgeon

Phase I: Introduction to da Vinci Technology:
- Test drive the da Vinci Surgical System
- Review procedure video relevant to your planned da Vinci procedures
- Complete live epicenter and/or standard case observation
- Complete live standard case observation

Phase II: da Vinci Technology Training:
- Complete da Vinci Technology online training (recommended)
- Complete da Vinci Technology In-Service with da Vinci representative
- Complete da Vinci Technology online assessment
- Perform da Vinci Technology Skills Drills
    - Skills Drills
    - Skills Simulator™ (if available)
- Review two full-length procedure videos relevant to your planned da Vinci procedures on da Vinci Online Community
- Complete preparation for da Vinci Technology Training (All above prerequisites must be complete prior to attendance).

In our experience with *da Vinci* Technology Training, increased retention, improvement of system skills and confidence are connected to the immediate application of the skills learned in *da Vinci* Technology Training. As a result, we highly recommend that the surgeon schedule at least two cases at his/her hospital to immediately following the *da Vinci* Technology Training.

Schedule and attend da Vinci Technology Training:

Important: da Vinci Technology Training is either 1 or 2 days, dependent on clinical specialty. Training times are dependent on the training center's hours of operation. Please contact your *da Vinci* representative for start and end times.
- If an attendee is more than 30 minutes late, the training may be cancelled and no certificate awarded.
- Leaving the training event prior to the completion of all tasks, will result in no certificate being awarded.

- The surgeon is responsible for all costs associated with rescheduling when the reschedule is due to tardiness or early departure.
- If the surgeon is unable to complete the protocol within the scheduled time, no certificate will be awarded; however, rescheduling to complete another full *da Vinci* Technology Training will be permitted at no cost to the surgeon.

In this phase, exercises which will allow the surgeon to obtain basic skills and become familiar with the 3D environment will be performed by trainee on simulator modules as well as porcine model. These are as follow:

1. Port placement, Instrument control
2. Camera control
3. Fourth arm control
4. Coordinate tool control
5. Ball placement
6. Spatial control
7. Needle handling
8. Basic electrocautery
9. Tissue cutting
10. Tissue retraction
11. Blunt tissue dissection
12. Vessel dissection
13. Knot tying.

Phase III: Initial Case Series Plan:

Complete initial case series: In our experience, a proctor provides important guided training in the early *da Vinci* cases. One role of a proctor is to guide the surgeon and his/her *da Vinci* Surgery team through their initial *da Vinci* cases to assist with their mastery of the technology. The proctor may also be required to provide an assessment of the surgeon's surgical skills with the *da Vinci* Surgical System to your hospital. Your hospital's requirements for proctoring will govern, as *intuitive* does not provide any credentials or privileges. In addition, the surgeon should consider additional proctoring if she/he determines that it would be beneficial to his/her practice. The surgeon should be proctored until she/he determines, in his/her surgical judgment that he/she is sufficiently competent to operate independently.

Complete two da Vinci Technology skills development activities per week:
- Assist in a *da Vinci* procedure
- Perform a *da Vinci* procedure
- Complete a *da Vinci* Technology Skills Drills session
- Complete a *da Vinci Skills Simulator* session (if available)
- Review a *da Vinci* Surgery procedure video relevant to your planned *da Vinci* procedures.

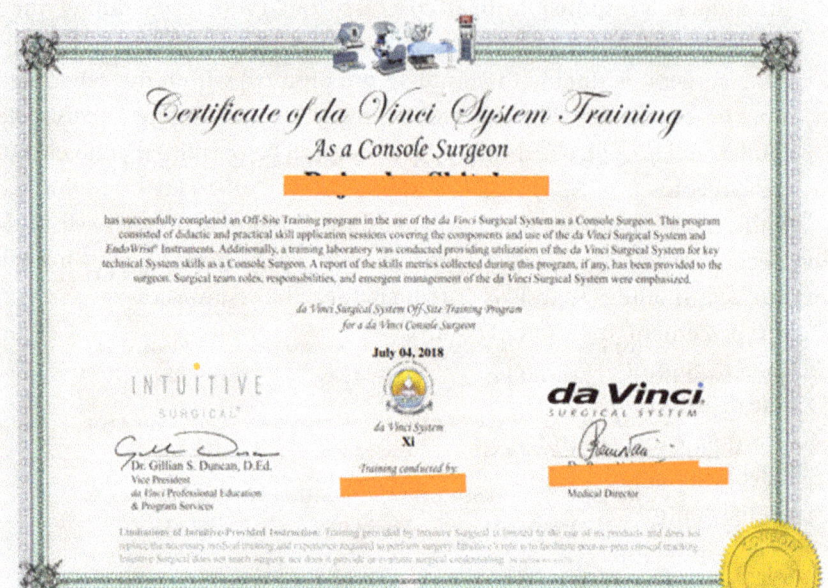

Fig. 4.2: Sample of *da Vinci* training certificate.

Phase IV: Continuing Development
- Attend surgeon-led course(s) (course details available in the da Vinci Training Passport brochure and course catalog. If not available in your market, please check with your da Vinci representative for course details.)
- Complete at least two additional activities after initial case series:
  - Surgeon lecture program
  - Complex *da Vinci* procedure observation
  - Complex *da Vinci* procedure video review
  - *da Vinci* surgery webinar
  - Peer-to-Peer consultation via Surgical Congress.

Certificate awarded at the end of completion of phase II (Fig. 4.2). After getting this certificate you are eligible to access console and do the surgeries.

Fellowships

Fellowships in robotic gynecology, robotic gyne-oncology are announced regularly by institutions on their websites where regular robotic surgeries are done and guides are available to train fellows. These are usually of 6 months to 1 year duration. Candidates can apply online and they will be called if selected depending on their publications, resume, and references. Fee structure and stipend varies depending on institution. The Vattikuti foundation is one which regularly announces national as well as international fellowships on their website *vfrsi.vattikutifoundation.com*. For other opportunities, you can search on google.com.

During training fellows will be trained thoroughly about technology of robots, port placement, docking, undocking, dissection methods, use of electrocautery in robotics, suturing techniques, complications and safety measures.

After completion of training fellows will be awarded fellowship certificate and can work at parent institutions or can grab opportunities available at other robotic centers.

Pay scales for robotic surgeons differ according to institutions and patient load as cost of consumables required for single surgery is also high. Surgeons usually get more paid for robotic surgeries as total cost of surgical procedure is also high.

After robotic training there is definite change in operative acumen due to 3D vision and EndoWrist movements. Over a period of time after performing substantial number of cases surgeon can go for more complicated cases, e.g. stage 3 and 4 endometriosis, radical hysterectomies, etc.

CHAPTER 5

Gynecological Oncology

Santhosh Kuriakose

PROLOGUE

"The unreturned envelope and the interview whose results were never announced."

My journey in pursuance of Gynecologic Oncology started in 2006 when I finished my postgraduate training in gynecology. I was particularly interested in undergoing fellowship program at a premier institution in India. I wrote a letter to them informing about my interest in pursuing Gynecologic Oncology. I waited hopefully, but the reply never came. Another premier institution in India announced its Gynecologic-Oncology fellowship program, I applied and was called for an interview. Alas! the results of the interview were never published in the website. At that time National Eligibility cum Entrance Test-Super Specialty (NEET)-SS was non-existent. Years later I joined a 2-year fellowship program at Amrita Institute of Medical Sciences, Kochi, Kerala, India which is now a *Master of Surgery (MCh) training center* in Kerala. I was the first trained Gynecologic Oncologist in our institution and started the first Gynecologic-Oncology Division in the Department of Obstetrics and Gynecology (OBG), which has completed 6 years. We have taken up Research Project with grant from Science and Engineering Research Board and the Indian Council of Medical Research (ICMR).

TRAINING OPPORTUNITIES IN GYNECOLOGIC ONCOLOGY IN INDIA

Role of a Gynecologic Oncologist

Every year cervical cancer affects 125,000 women in India and 75,000 deaths occurs due to the disease. Cervical cancer is ranked as the second and ovarian cancer the fourth among the top cancers affecting women in India. (The top five cancers among women in India—breast, cervix, colorectum, ovary and lip, oral cavity) The number of cancer cases is increasing every year and the burden of cancer treatment is likely to increase in the coming years.

It has long been recognized that clinical and oncological outcome of gynecological cancers are best with treatment in the hands of a Gynecologic Oncologist.[1-3] Most of international guidelines such as National

Comprehensive Cancer Network (NCCN) and the American Society of Clinical Oncology (ASCO) recommend involvement by a Gynecologic Oncologist. The American College of Obstetricians and Gynecologists (ACOG) defines Gynecologic Oncologist as "a specialist in obstetrics and gynecology who is prepared to provide consultation on comprehensive management of patients with gynecologic cancer and who works in an institutional setting wherein all the effective forms of cancer therapy are available".[4] The importance of this specialty has percolated into Indian scenarios as well. The management protocols of gynecological cancers specify specialized procedures, most of which, can be undertaken only after specialized training. Besides the training will give great surgical perspective and outlook that the skills acquired will be of great use in tackling difficult cases in gynecology and obstetrics.

Training Programs—MCh in Gynecologic Oncology

When we look at the opportunity for Gynecologic Oncology training in India, the major shift that has occurred is the NEET Superspecialty entrance examinations. The basic qualification for applying for the course is MD/MS/DNB in OBG. The information can be obtained from the official website of Medical Council of India https://www.mciindia.org/CMS/information-desk/college-and-course-search (Table 5.1).

MCI recognition status of these MCh seats are subject to variation and the reader is advised to verify the current status by clicking the "Recognized"

Table 5.1: Number of MCh seats available all over India at different universities.

S. No.	Institution	University	Number of seats
1.	Tata Memorial Center, Mumbai, Maharashtra	Homi Bhabha National Institute (Deemed University)	2
2.	Kidwai Memorial Institute of Oncology, Bengaluru, Karnataka	Rajiv Gandhi University of Health Sciences	1
3.	St. John's Medical College, Bengaluru, Karnataka	Rajiv Gandhi University of Health Sciences	1
4.	Amrita School of Medicine, Kochi, Kerala	Amrita Vishwa Vidyapeetham University (Deemed)	2
5.	BJ Medical College, Ahmedabad, Gujarat	Gujarat University	1
6.	Acharya Harihar RCC, Cuttack, Odisha	Utkal University	2
7.	Christian Medical College, Vellore, Tamil Nadu	The Tamil Nadu Dr. MGR Medical University	2

status in the mentioned MCI site. Some of the seats are categorized under *private* and hence admissions to the seats are as per the policy of the respective institutions.

All admissions are done through the NEET-SS entrance examination. NEET-SS is a single window entrance examination for all Super Specialty DM/MCh courses in India. No other entrance examination, either at state or institution level, shall be valid for entry to DM/MCh courses as per the Indian Medical Council (Amendment) Act, 2016 wef 2017 admission session. It is mandatory to qualify NEET-SS examination for gaining entry to MCh.

The information is available in the website of National Board of Examinations *http://examarchive.natboard.edu.in/neetss/ index.html*. The details of NEET-SS are available at: *http://examarchive.natboard.edu.in/neetss/list-dm-mch-courses-neetss-2017.html*.

NEET-SS examination is conducted once a year usually in the months of June or July which is followed by a strictly merit-based centralized online counseling conducted by the Directorate General of Health Services, Ministry of Health and Family Welfare. Seats are allotted via this counseling process, so as to commence classes in August of that year.

NEET-SS Examination Pattern 2018

Forty percent of the questions shall be from the feeder broad specialty course and the remaining 60% shall be from the superspecialty course selected by the candidate at the time online submission of application form. There shall be a separate question paper for each superspecialty course/clubbed group. The total number of questions in each question paper shall be 100 which shall be divided into two parts: (1) Part A and (2) Part B. All the questions shall be postgraduate (PG) exit level. The examination pattern of NEET-SS 2018 will be as follows:
- *Question paper:* Part A will have 40 questions and Part B will have 60 questions. Time allocated will be 45 minutes and 60 minutes for Part A and B, respectively.
- *Marking scheme* for NEET-SS will be as follows: 4 marks should be allocated for the correct response and 1 mark shall be deducted for incorrect answer. Zero marks should be allocated for the unattempted questions.

These patterns may vary every year and the aspirant is advised to check the website for any changes.

MCh Seats at All India Institute of Medical Sciences

All India Institute of Medical Sciences (AIIMS) conducts separate examinations for the MCh courses for AIIMS, New Delhi and AIIMS, Rishikesh (Uttarakhand). In the January examination, admission will be done for 1 open seat and

Table 5.2: MCh seats at All India Institute of Medical Sciences (New Delhi and Rishikesh).

AIIMS Seats	Hospital	Seats
1.	AIIMS, New Delhi	3 seats
2.	AIIMS, Rishikesh	1 seat

1 sponsored seat at AIIMS, New Delhi. During the July examination session, admission will be done for 1 open seat at AIIMS, New Delhi and 1 open seat at AIIMS, Rishikesh (Table 5.2).

Hence, the total number of MCh seats in India is currently 15; 11 through NEET-SS and 4 by AIIMS entrance examination.

Further it may be noted that all who have a MD/MS/DNB in Gynecology are eligible to apply for MCh in Surgical Oncology through NEET-SS examinations. The numbers of MCh Surgical Oncology seats per year are 88 across India.

Gynecologic Oncology Fellowship Programs in India

Considering the limited number of MCh seats available in India it is very clear that majority of aspirants will have the option of doing 2 years Fellowship Programs available in the Institutions across India. The MCI has specified the basic Academic qualifications for teaching faculty in a Surgical Oncology Department to be MCh (Surgical Oncology)/MS (Surgery) or MS (ENT) or MS (Orthopedics) or MD (OBG) with 2 years special training in Surgical Oncology. A DNB qualified candidate in broad specialty will be considered equivalent to MS/MS (see *https://old.mciindia.org/Rules-and-Regulation/Teachers-Eligibility-Qualifications-Regulations-1998.pdf*). Hence, a 2-year Fellowship program can be considered for acquiring necessary skills. At the same time it should be very clear that Fellowships are not recognized by MCI as an accepted training program. The institutions providing fellowships in India are listed in Table 5.3 and are liable to vary every year.

AIMS AND OBJECTIVES OF TRAINING PROGRAMS

Course is intended to give exposure and training in all major gynecologic-oncologic procedures. Multidisciplinary care is the core of optimal patient care. The candidate should get a clear concept of overall management of a gynecological cancer case, by involving the radiation oncologist, medical oncologist, palliative care specialists and pathologists in all patients and in some cases other specialists. The candidate should understand the advantage of minimally invasive surgery (MIS) and have a discernment of its use. They will be trained in community oncology and community intervention strategies since the field of preventive oncology have advanced and India

Table 5.3: The Fellowship in MCh available at different institutes in India.

S. No.	Institution	Period	Type
1.	Regional Cancer Centre, Thiruvananthapuram, Kerala http://www.rcctvm.org	2 years	Institutional Fellowship
2.	Malabar Cancer Centre, Thalassery, Kerala http://mcc.kerala.gov.in	1 year	Institutional Fellowship
3.	Tata Memorial Hospital, Kolkata, West Bengal	2 years	Institutional Fellowship
4.	CMC Vellore, Tamil Nadu	2 years	Institutional Fellowship
5.	Dr Bhubaneswar Borooah Cancer Institute (BBCI), Guwahati, Assam	2 years	Institutional Fellowship
6.	Lakeshore Hospital, Kochi, Kerala http://www.vpslakeshorehospital.com/courses-offered	2 years	AGOI Fellowship
7.	Action Cancer Hospital, Delhi	2 years	AGOI Fellowship
8.	Fortis Memorial Institute, Gurugram, Haryana	2 years	AGOI Fellowship
9	Rajiv Gandhi Cancer Institute and Research Centre, Delhi http://www.rgcirc.org/academics/fellowship/	1 year	IMA AMS fellowship

is yet to use this potential to its full benefit. He/she should have a spirit of "lifelong learner" with an eagerness to do research whose results need to be disseminated through publications.

At the end of the training the candidate should be confident of doing procedures such as radical hysterectomy, staging laparotomy for Ca ovary and endometrium, ilioinguinal block dissection, para-aortic lymph node dissection and pelvic exenteration. He/she should be familiar with the commonly used techniques of radiotherapy for treating gynecologic malignancy (including brachytherapy, planning of external RT treatment and execution) and their side effects and also regarding commonly used chemotherapy schedules. He/she should be capable of delivering palliative care by alleviate pain and other symptoms associated with advanced gynecologic malignancies while also addressing the patients' social, emotional and spiritual needs. He/she should be well versed with community aspects of cancer screening including cancer registry, familiar with all aspects of preventive oncology, be able to conduct screening, early detection and health awareness campaigns. The candidate should also be competent to plan and implement community intervention strategies and be trained to link up with the existing healthcare system.

GYNECOLOGIC ONCOLOGY FELLOWSHIPS ABROAD

Fellowship programs are available in countries such as USA, Canada and UK. To apply for Gynecologic Oncology Fellowship programs in United States of America,[4] the applicants must have completed USMLE Steps 1, 2CK, and 2CS have ECFMG certification. On a broad scale, they will have to complete the equivalent of UG and PG before applying for the Fellowship programs abroad.

CONCLUSION

Gynecologic malignancies as a group constitute the most common malignancy among females in India. Most patients with gynecologic malignancies would first go to a gynecologist and be guided by them regarding their management. India requires a large number of Gynecologists to be exposed to gynecologic oncology so that We would be fully equipped to take correct decisions regarding management of gynecologic malignancies and also take up leadership and become involved in policy decisions at the National and International platforms that will provide better health to our women.

REFERENCES

1. Vernooij F, Heintz P, Witteveen E, et al. The outcomes of ovarian cancer treatment are better when provided by gynecologic oncologists and in specialized hospitals: a systematic review. Gynecol Oncol. 2007;105(3):801-12.
2. du Bois A, Rochon J, Pfisterer J, et al. Variations in institutional infrastructure, physician specialization and experience, and outcome in ovarian cancer: a systematic review. Gynecol Oncol. 2009;112(2):422-36.
3. Fung-Kee-Fung M, Kennedy EB, Biagi J, et al. The optimal organization of gynecologic oncology services: a systematic review. Curr Oncol. 2015;22(4):e282-93.
4. American Board of Obstetrics and Gynecology. (2015). Guidelines. [online] Available from http://www.abog.org/publications. [Accessed November, 2018].

CHAPTER 6

Fetal Medicine

Vivek Krishnan

INTRODUCTION

Fetal medicine is a relatively young subspecialty in obstetrics. Therefore, the fact that there is room for a lot more specialists not withstanding, there is a shortage of quality training programs in this field. The few centers that offer training have long waiting lists of applicants. Nevertheless, planning ahead of time and a focused intent to subspecialize in fetal medicine after postgraduation can help students secure the training program they desire. This is where a thorough understanding of the various available training programs in India and abroad comes in handy.

Before deciding which program to choose, two crucial questions are to be answered:

1. Do you intend to be a full-time Fetal Medicine/Maternal Fetal Medicine (MFM/Perinatology) specialist or an Obstetrician with a basic understanding of obstetric ultrasound and fetal medicine?

    If it is the former, it is important to choose programs that offer a longer duration of training (longer the better).

2. Where do you plan to work after training—India or abroad?

    Unless there are plans to work and settle abroad, it makes no sense to pursue foreign programs as most of these would require additional steps to become board certified and/or council registered in respective countries. These consume time, effort and money. Moreover, hands on exposure would be limited in most foreign programs because they cater to a lot less number of pregnant women than most Indian programs do. Some of the programs being offered in our country are at par with most international programs, if not better and are a lot more reasonably priced too.

    Table 6.1 shows basic information on various training programs available in India. Further details on each of these may be obtained by visiting the respective links thereof.

Chapter 6: Fetal Medicine 43

Table 6.1: Basic information on various medical training programs available in India on fetal medicine.

S. No	Institution	Course offered	Qualification	Duration	Selection	Intake	Contact
1.	Adi's Advanced Fetal Care Centre	Fetal Medicine Fellowship	PG in Obstetrics/ Radiology	6 months	Personal interview	6 trainees/batch in January and July	Dr Adi Narayan Makkam info@adifetalmedicine.com +91-7090380000
2.	AIIMS, New Delhi	Fellowship in Maternal Fetal Medicine	MD/MS/DNB Obstetrics and Gynecology + Senior Residency for 3 years	1 year	Entrance examination followed by personal interview	2 (Usually July session)	Dr Dipika Deka http://dm.aiimsexams.org/ProspectusEligibility.html
3.	Amrita Institute of Medical Sciences, Kochi	Post-Doctoral Fellowship in Fetal Medicine	MD/MS/DNB OBG	2 years	Personal interview	1 seat	Dr Vivek Krishnan www.aimshospital.org perinatology@aims.amrita.edu +91-484-2851088
		Fellowship in Advanced Obstetric Ultrasound and Fetal ECHO	MD/MS/DNB OBG or Radiology	1 year	Personal interview	1 seat	
		Fellowship in Basic Obstetric Ultrasound	MD/MS/DNB OBG or Radiology	6 months	Personal interview	2 seats	
4.	Ansh Fetal Care Centre, Ahmedabad	Fellowship in Fetal Medicine/ Advanced OBG Ultrasound	MD/MS/DNB/DGO MD/DNB/DMRD Radiology	6 months/ 1 year	Personal interview	1 seat	Dr Janak Desai anshfetalcare@gmail.com 079-26584777

Contd...

Contd...

S. No	Institution	Course offered	Qualification	Duration	Selection	Intake	Contact
5.	Apollo Centre for Fetal Medicine, Apollo Indraprastha Hospital, New Delhi	FMF–ACFM-FOGSI Fellowship in Fetomaternal Medicine	MD/MS/DNB Obstetrics and Gynecology	4 years	Personal interview	1 seat	Dr Anita Kaul http://www.fetalmedicineindia.in/011-29873018
		ACFM Fellowship in Fetomaternal Medicine	MD/MS/DNB Obstetrics and Gynecology	2 years	Personal interview	2 seats	
6.	Bangalore Fetal Medicine Centre	Fetal Medicine Fellowship	MD/MS/DNB/DGO in Obstetrics and Gynecology	2 years	Personal interview	Jan, April, July, October intake 2 seats/quarter	Dr Prathima Radhakrishnan http://www.bangalorefetalmedicine.com 9945813170
		Fellowship in Obstetric Ultrasound	MD/MS/DNB/DGO in Obstetrics and Gynecology	1 year	Personal interview	Jan, April, July, October intake 1 seat/quarter	
7.	Bangalore RCOG Trust (The Rangadore Memorial Hospital)	Fellowship in Fetomaternal Medicine	MD/MS (OBG)/ DNB/MRCOG/DGO	18 months	Personal interview	–	blorercog@gmail.com ssspt.rmh6@gmail.com +91 80 2656 1724
8.	Chikitsa Diagnostic and Ultrasound Training Centre, Mumbai	Fellowship in Obstetric Ultrasound	MD/MS/DNB/ in Obstetrics and Gynecology or Radiology	6 months and 1 year	Personal interview	–	Dr Anirudh Badade Dr Meenakshi Badade +91 9987115680 Chikitsa1995@gmail.com

Contd...

Contd...

S. No	Institution	Course offered	Qualification	Duration	Selection	Intake	Contact
9.	CIMAR Kochi/ Edappal	Fellowship in Fetomaternal Medicine	MD/MS/DNB/DGO in Obstetrics and Gynecology	1 year	Personal interview	Cochin and Edappal Centres, 2 batches in January and July 2 seats per batch	Dr Meenu Batra Dr Bijoy Balakrishnan cimarindia.org cimarcochin@gmail.com +91 484 4134444
		Advanced OBGYN Ultrasound Course	MD/DNB/DMRD (Radiology)	6 months	Personal interview		
		Fellowship in Fetal Medicine	MD/MS/DNB/DGO (OBG)/MD/DNB/ DMRD (Radiology)	2 years	Personal interview	2 seats January intake	Dr Suseela Vavilala Dr Geeta Kolar academics@fernandezhospital.com +91 - 8008902042 04041411215
10.	Fernandez Hospital, Hyderabad	Fellowship in Obstetric Ultrasound	MD/MS/DNB/DGO (OBG)/MD/DNB/ DMRD (Radiology)	1 year	Personal interview	2 seats in Jan 2 seats in July	
		Advanced Ultrasound Course in Obstetrics	MD/MS/DNB (OBG)	6 months	Personal interview	Jan, April, July, October intake 2 seats/quarter	
11	IIRRH, Bangalore	Certification Course in Obstetric Ultrasound	MS/DGO/DNB (OBG)/MD/DNB (Radiology)/DMRD	6 months	Written Exam (MCQ) followed by interview	-	Dr BS Ramamurthy +91 7829 192444 info.iirrh@gmail.com

Contd...

Contd...

S. No	Institution	Course offered	Qualification	Duration	Selection	Intake	Contact
12.	MEDISCAN, Chennai	Fellowship in Fetal Medicine	MS(OG)/MD(OG)/ DNB(OG)/MRCOG	3 years	Personal interview	8 seats, 4 each in January/July	Prof. S Suresh Dr Indrani Suresh www.mediscansystems.org
		Fellowship in Advanced Obstetric and Gynec Ultrasound	Obstetricians and Radiologists	1 year	Personal interview	16 seats 4 each in Jan, April, July, Oct	
		Fellowship in Obstetric Ultrasound	Obstetricians and Radiologists	6 months	Personal interview	8 seats 4 each in April and October	+91 90940 21675
13.	Navodaya Resolution Fetal Medicine Centre, Hyderabad	Fetal Medicine Fellowship	MD/MS/DNB/DGO in Obstetrics and Gynecology	1 year	Personal interview	2 seats July intake	Dr Chinmayee Ratha info@resolutionfetalcare.com +91-9885348600
14.	National Board of Examination	FNB in High Risk Pregnancy and Perinatology	MD/MS/DNB Obstetrics and Gynecology	2 years	Fellowship Entrance Examination	(MAMC), New Delhi-2 Safdarjang Hospital and VMMC, New Delhi-2 Edappal Hospital, Malapuram, Kerala-2 Fernandez Hospital, Hyderabad-4 Kamineni Hospital, Hyderabad-2	http://www.natboard.edu.in

Contd...

Contd...

S. No	Institution	Course offered	Qualification	Duration	Selection	Intake	Contact
15.	Nethra Scans Fetal Medicine Centre, Tiruppur	Fellowship in Fetal Medicine	MD/MS/DNB/ in Obstetrics and Gynecology or Radiology	1 year	Personal interview	1 seat July intake	Dr P Devarajan drdevabir@gmail.com +91 9787913402 www.nethrascanstirupur.org/
16.	Paras Advanced Centre for Fetal Medicine, Ahmedabad	Fellowship in Fetal Medicine	MD/MS/DNB/ in Obstetrics and Gynecology or Radiology	6 months	Personal interview	2 seats	Dr Prashant Acharya www.parasfetalmedicine.com 097277 86079
		Certificate Course in Fetal Medicine (ICOG)	MD/MS/DNB/ in Obstetrics and Gynecology	6 months	Personal interview (Apply through ICOG site)	2 seats	
17.	Ria Clinic, Mumbai						Dr Chander Lulla riaclinic@gmail.com 9833938025
18.	SONOSCAN, Coimbatore	Fellowship in Advanced Sonography in Obstetrics, Gynecology and Fetal Medicine	MS (OG), MD (OG), DGO, DNB (OG)/ MD (RD), DMRD, DNB (RD)	1 year	Personal interview	-	Dr Boopathy Vijayaraghavan sonoscanscr@gmail.com or radhika@sonoscan.in 0422-2477484

Contd...

Contd...

S. No	Institution	Course offered	Qualification	Duration	Selection	Intake	Contact
19.	SRMC, Chennai	Fellowship in Fetal Medicine	MD (OB-GYN)/DNB (OB-GYN)/DGO/ MDRD/DMRD/DNB (Radiology)	2 years	Personal interview	2 seats January intake	Dr Chitra Andrew www.sriramachandra.edu.in
		Fellowship in Advanced Ultrasound in Obstetrics and Gynecology	MD (OB-GYN)/DNB (OB-GYN)/DGO/ MDRD/DMRD/DNB (Radiology)	1 year	Personal interview	2 seats Jan/July	
		Fellowship in Basic Ultrasound in Obstetrics and Gynecology	MD (OB-GYN)/DNB (OB-GYN)/DGO/ MDRD/DMRD/DNB (Radiology)	6 months	Personal interview	3 seats Jan/July	
20.	Thane Ultrasound Centre	Fellowship in Women's Imaging (DY Patil University)	MD/DNB (Radiodiagnosis) DMRD + 1 year	1 year	Merit based interview	1 seat (March intake)	Dr Nitin Chaubal Dr Jyoti Chaubal
	VS Hospital, NHL Municipal Medical College, Ahmedabad	Fellowship in Fetal Medicine	MS (OBG)	1 year	Personal interview	1 seat	Dr Janak Desai
21.		Fellowship in Advanced Ultrasonography (Obs and Gynec)	MS/DGO/Equivalent MD Radiology/ DMRD/ Equivalent	6 months	Personal interview	3 seats	www.nhlmmc.edu.in/ dean_nhlmmc@yahoo.co.in (079) 26578452, 26576275
22.	Women's Centre, Coimbatore	Fellowship in Maternal-Fetal Medicine	MS/MD/DNB (OG) MS/DNB (Radio Diagnosis)	2 years	Personal interview	2 seats July intake	www.womenscenterindia.com info@womenscenterindia.com 0422 4201000

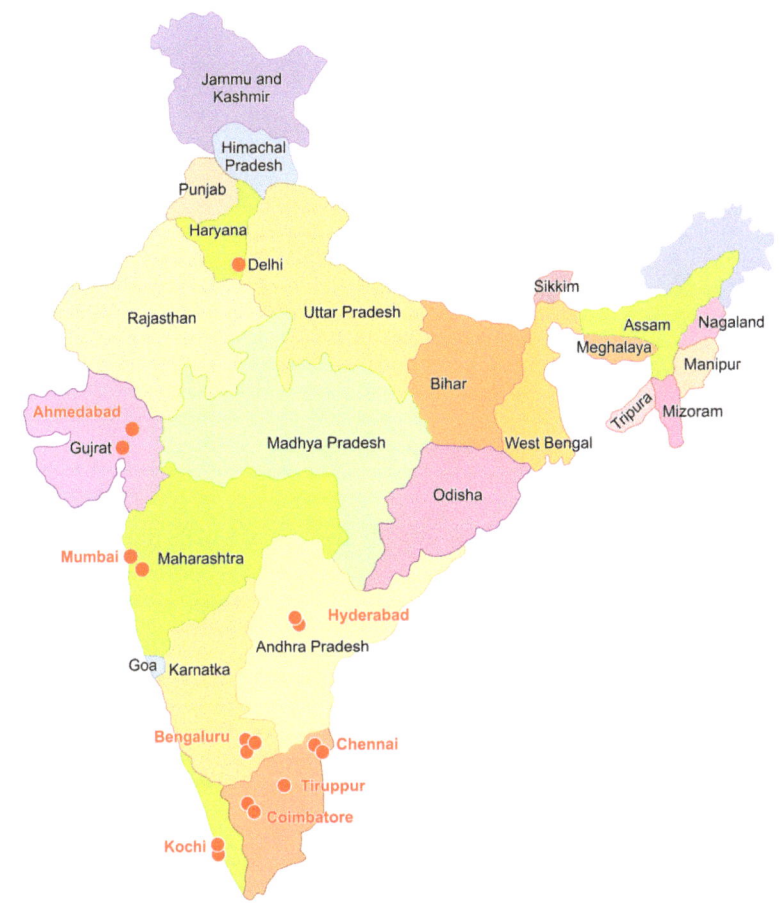

Fig. 6.1: Map of fellowship programs in India.

FOREIGN PROGRAMS

When it comes to foreign programs, there are number of short-term courses and a few long-term ones, but very few that are actually foreign graduate friendly. We have listed a hand-picked few which we feel may be feasible for a postgraduate from India (Figs. 6.1 and 6.2).

United States

There are close to 80 centers offering Maternal-Fetal medicine fellowships in the United States, but mostly to specialists certified by the American Board. While matching to these courses is similar to the match process for residency, there are several key differences you need to know about to successfully navigate the process. Applying for fellowship is expensive, stressful, and time consuming. According to a 2016 article most applicants spend more than

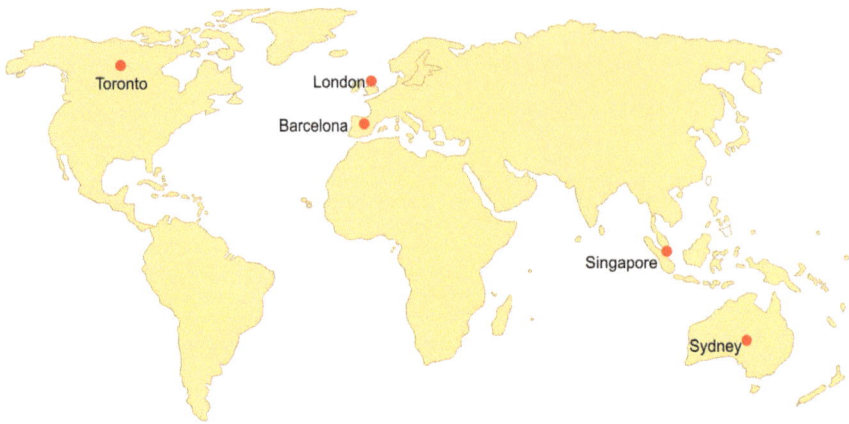

Fig. 6.2: Map of international fellowship programs.

10 days away on interviews and spend an average of $5,286 during the interview season.

Applications are through ERAS (Electronic Residency Application Service) and are to be made online where you would be required to submit your curriculum vitae (CV) and 3-4 letter of recommendation.

The important links are:
- *https://www.smfm.org/fellowships*
- *https://s3.amazonaws.com/cdn.smfm.org/media/1551/Fellowship_at_a_Glance_Updated_July112018.xlsx.*

Europe

In UK the fellowships are offered in the NHS hospitals.

The usual pathway is after completing MRCOG (Membership of Royal College of Obstetricians and Gynaecologists—ST 5) and then entering ST6-7 (2 years) and getting CCST (Certificate of Completion in Specialist Training) in Maternal Fetal Medicine (MFM). For overseas candidates, one has to clear MRCOG, work as Registrar in UK and then apply for specialist training in MFM.

Fetal medicine fellowships are offered by the Fetal Medicine Foundation (FMF) UK, for UK and overseas candidates. For this one has to complete MD/MS in OBG and then apply via the Fetal Medicine Foundation (FMF) UK website. The selection criteria are not explicit, but depend on their requirement for research fellows and VISAs they can offer.

There are also the RCOG Diploma programs in ultrasound. The details are available in the RCOG website.

Link: fellowship@fetalmedicine.org

In other European countries, it is difficult to obtain MFM fellowships. The University of Barcelona offers Master program in MFM for consultants with at least 2 years' experience in MFM. The details can be obtained from the MFM website of the University of Barcelona. (*http://medicinafetalbarcelona.org/docencia2/en/Curso/evento-internacional/international-master-maternal-fetal-medicine*)

Australia/New Zealand

The Royal Australian and New Zealand College of Obstetricians and Gynaecologists (RANZCOG) subspecialist training programs are offered in
- Certification in Maternal and Fetal Medicine (CMFM)
- Certification in Obstetrical and Gynaecological Ultrasound (COGU).

These are 3 years full-time subspecialist training in a prospectively approved subspecialty training position.

Eligibility

- International Subspecialists who hold a recognized international subspecialist qualification from a recognized college or national certifying body may apply to the college for assessment for recognition as an International Subspecialist.
- Applications will initially be assessed by the RANZCOG Specialist International Medical Graduate (SIMG) Assessment Committee.
- Eligible applications will be referred to the relevant Subspecialty Committee.
- Eligible candidates to enter the relevant SIMG Subspecialist pathway to Fellowship and Subspecialist Certification.
- *Link:* https://www.ranzcog.edu.au/Training/Subspecialist-Training.

Singapore

The National University of Health Singapore and the KK Women's and Children's Hospital offer honorary Fellowship to Foreign graduates. These are self-sponsored programs. Eligibility criteria include IELTS/TOEFL, age less than 35 years and 3 years post-House surgeon experience. Interested candidates may apply directly with CV, and 2 referral letters.

Canada

The University of Toronto and Mount Sinai Hospital offers a 2-year fellowship in Maternal Fetal Medicine. If you are not a Canadian citizen or permanent resident, you will be required to pay the Work Permit Processing fee ($150.00 CND) along with the Fellowship Application Form. Candidates have to contact the course directors directly to apply. Application deadline for International Medical Graduates is July 1st, two (2) years preceding the year of your anticipated start date. A valid TOEFL IBT score, cover letter, and academic CV are required.

Initial enquiries for the Maternal Fetal Medicine Fellowship training program should be directed to *mfmfellowship.MSH@sinaihealthsystem.ca*. Forward CV as well as a cover letter explaining your interest in MFM training as well as your interest in the specific program. If you fulfill their entry requirements, you will be asked to complete a Fellowship Application Form. You will need to provide three written, electronically-signed PDF, or faxed references. *(https://www.obgyn.utoronto.ca/maternal-fetal-medicinercpsc)*

Wishing you a wonderful career in Fetal Medicine!

CHAPTER 7

High-risk Pregnancy and Perinatology

Raymond George

WHAT ARE THE OPTIONS FOR HIGH-RISK PREGNANCY AND PERINATOLOGY?

The concept of subspecialization arises from the fact that it is impossible for an individual to master in depth all or even most areas of a subject. So a high degree of specialization ensures proper special training, experience and skills which improve the knowledge, practice, teaching and research. As a new speciality, high-risk pregnancy and perinatology is a subspecialization in obstetrics and gynecology dedicated to the optimization of pregnancy and perinatal outcome.[1] The subspeciality is well established in the west long before. The Royal College of Obstetricians and Gynaecologists (RCOG) and American College of Obstetricians and Gynecologists (ACOG) have fellowship programs for the last 25 years. There are around 25 training centers in UK and Ireland which is approved by RCOG.

As a speciality maternal-fetal-medicine (MFM)/high-risk pregnancy and perinatology is a relatively a novel concept for the medical fraternity in India. It is more than 10 years since National Board of Examination have initiated the training of this speciality through a 2 years fellowship program. Till now there are only very few centers which has such an ongoing program in this speciality. This is a major obstacle in its outreach among people.

The leading hypothesis such as Pedersen hypothesis (fetal hyperinsulinemia), the Frenkel hypothesis (fuel mediated teratogenesis), Barker's hypothesis (fetal origin of adult disease) and the inverted pyramid of pregnancy care by Sir Nicolaides hypothesis and the current research's demonstrate the strong interconnection between the maternal (M) and the fetal (F) components of the MFM speciality.[2]

With evolution of MFM speciality many of the women with chronic health diseases, for whom pregnancy was previously considered an absolute contraindication has a ray of hope to conceive under the guidance of these specialists. In many cases where an obstetrician will advise termination in view of the high risk for the mother, the MFM specialist may be able to help them through a proper pre-pregnancy counseling, continuous monitoring throughout pregnancy in collaboration with the concerned multidisciplinary team. There are a lot of implications in such high-risk pregnancies starting

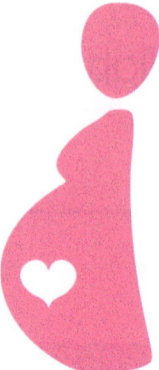

Fig. 7.1: High-risk Pregnancy: Care for both

from the pre-pregnancy counseling the complication to the mother as well as the fetus, the drugs used, intrapartum and postpartum management are considered (Fig. 7.1).

IS IT A DEGREE OR A FELLOWSHIP?

The only available training program in India is the fellowship program offered by the National Board of Examinations. This FNBE (fellowship of National Board of Examinations) program is a 2-year course. Presently there are six seats all over India across three centers which gives comprehensive training in maternal and fetal medicine, which includes Nuchal translucency (NT) certification from the FMF (fetal medicine foundation).

HOW TO APPLY/PREPARE?

National board of examinations conducts yearly fellowship entrance examinations for the subspecialties in obstetrics and gynecology including reproductive medicine/high-risk pregnancy and perinatology as a single paper. It is conducted in the month of January followed by centralized counseling at New Delhi. There will be total 130 questions which will be of multiple choice and objective in nature with single correct response out of the 130 questions, 100 questions are from obstetrics and gynecology and 30 marks is from medical genetics (which is optional). Duration of the exam is 2 hours. Each question will carry one mark and maximum mark is 100. There is no negative mark for a given question. Candidates who get 50% will be considered qualified. The answers have to be given in OMR sheet. The marks obtained in obstetrics and gynecology component (i.e. out of 100) shall be scaled to 180 and a common merit list shall be prepared (based on performance in 180 + 30 = 210 questions) amongst all the eligible candidates from obstetrics and gynecology and candidates from medicine and pediatrics appearing in DNBCET-SS. Medical genetics is a 3-year superspeciality fellowship program for which there is a separate entrance exam for pediatrics and general medicine graduates. There will be a common questions for reproductive medicine/high-risk pregnancy and perinatology and allotment of the speciality shall be done at time of counseling.

Questions are based on the candidates' knowledge in the obstetrics and gynecology. It is advisable to refer the last 5 years of NEET PG question papers along with topics related to high risk pregnancy, reproductive medicine and medical genetics.

CONTENT TAUGHT IN THE FELLOWSHIP PROGRAM

In the 2-year fellowship program, a trainee should get a complete exposure in maternal medicine and fetal medicine focusing on the following areas.

Maternal Medicine

1. Pregnancy in women with chronic health issues.
2. Disease specific management of medical and surgical disorders of pregnancy.
3. Pre-pregnancy counseling for genetic disorders, bad obstetric history, high-risk pregnancy.
4. High-risk pregnancy outpatient services including combined clinics for specific medical disorders in pregnancy, multiple pregnancies, artificial reproductive technique related pregnancy.
5. Intensive care and high dependency unit management of complicated pregnancies.
6. Protocol-based management.
7. Postpartum and family planning clinics.
8. Audit/research-related activities.
9. Attending maternal near miss and mortality meeting.
10. Teaching/training of undergraduates and midwife.

Fetal Medicine

Hands on training in:
1. Early pregnancy ultrasound.
2. Aneuploidy screening.
3. Targeted imaging for fetal anomalies (TIFFA).
4. Prenatal invasive diagnostic procedures like chorionic villus sampling and amniocentesis.
5. Growth scans
6. Fetal autopsies.
7. Audit/research related activities
8. Neonatology and anesthesia postings.

What are the Opportunities after the Course?

Maternal fetal medicine is a brand new speciality with a lot of opportunities. As mentioned earlier it always better to take care both mother and fetus together. It is always a team approach when dealing with a pregnancy in women with chronic medical disorders. MFM specialist has a major role to play as the primary consultant in decision making throughout the pregnancy and postpartum care. He/She has to work in hand-in-hand with the other specialist in the multidisciplinary team.

As a relatively new speciality in India, opportunities will be scare initially and can be a challenge for the newly trained doctors. But there is always a hope that like many other subspecialties in medicine, this branch will also grow over time.

Unfortunately for various reasons the focus of maternal and fetal medicine subspecialty has been shifted over the past years to fetal medicine/ultrasound.[3] A combined approach of both components with equal importance is going to make this scenario much better.

REFERENCES

1. Farquharson DI. Review of subspeciality training in obstetrics and gynaecology. Best Pract Res Clin Obstet Gynaecol. 2010;24(6):721-9.
2. Cabero Roura L, Hod M. Identification, prevention, and monitoring of the "great obstetrical syndromes". Best Pract Res Clin Obstet Gynaecol. 2015;29(2):145-9.
3. Hod M, Lieberman N. Maternal-fetal medicine-how can we practically connect the "M" to the "F"? Best Pract Res Clin Obstet Gynaecol. 2015;29(2):270-83.

CHAPTER 8

MCh (Reproductive Medicine and Surgery)

Fessy Louis T, Aparna N, Ramesh P

INTRODUCTION

Obstetrics and gynecology (OBGYN) was considered as an end speciality branch for long time, as no further Medical Council of India (MCI) recognized subspecialty courses were available after MD/MS/DNB OBGYN. Many institutions offer fellowship program of duration from 15 days to 2 years, many of which are not recognized by any university. However, such recognition is not mandated as of now because you just need to do the work and you can start your own practice.

The National Board of Examinations (NBE) is running a postdoctoral fellowship (subspecialty) course named FNB (Fellow in NBE). The course started many years back and is currently having seats distributed all over India. The FNB courses under the specialty of OBGYN are FNB Reproductive Medicine (around 20 seats) and FNB High-risk pregnancy and Perinatology (around 8 seats). The admission is through an exam conducted by NBE (FAT: Fellowship admission test). It is usually conducted in the month of January-February every year and the applications are called for around November. The details are available in NBE website—www.nbe.edu, www.natboard.com.

But in the recent years the things have changed drastically and few superspeciality courses have been started which are recognized under MCI. One among them is MCh Reproductive Medicine and Surgery. It is a degree course of 3 years duration like any other MCh course recognized by MCI.

MCH REPRODUCTIVE MEDICINE AND SURGERY

Currently offered by only two institutions in India: (1) Sri Ramachandra Medical College (SRMC) Chennai and (2) Amrita Institute of Medical Sciences (AIMS), Kochi.

All India Institutes of Medical Sciences (AIIMS), New Delhi also now offers DM in reproductive medicine from 2017 onwards.

This specialty is a new one started initially in 2012 in SRMC. Amrita Institute of Medical Sciences, Kochi started this course in 2016 and both the colleges offer 2 seats per year.

The admission to SRMC and Amrita Hospital is through National Eligibility cum Entrance Test for Super Specialty (NEET-SS)—All India examination conducted every year in June-July period. The application is usually called for in the month of April-May every year. It is conducted by NBE, New Delhi through a computer-based test with testing centers all over India. The detailed process of examination is available in the website of NBE: www.nbe.edu.in.

Sri Aurobindo Institute of Medical Sciences (SAIMS), Indore also had DM reproductive medicine course until 2016, but has been discontinued from 2017 NEET-SS admission.

HOW TO APPLY/PREPARE FOR MCH REPRODUCTIVE MEDICINE AND SURGERY?

Application

National Eligibility cum Entrance Test for Super Specialty exam is an All India single entrance examination conducted by NBE, New Delhi for superspeciality courses, first started in June 2017.

It is a *boon* for all those who aspire to do further subspeciality in their respective specialities as a single entrance is made for all the seats available in India under one roof.

After MS/DNB OBGYN now we can think of doing a recognized superspeciality course like other specialities by getting through an entrance exam, which was not available for us earlier.

NEET-SS is an online examination conducted once in a year in June-July period with exam centers all over India. Presently you can opt for two superspecialities of your choice and the exam paper contains 40 questions of basic speciality and 60 questions each of particular superspeciality opted.

Preparation for MCh Reproductive Medicine

(The books which we read/referred are mentioned here. It is always of your choice with what books you find comfortable to read.)

Books read during MS/DNB OBGYN postgraduation is the hard core to be revised: Williams Obstetrics, Novak Gynecology, Ian Donald Obstetrics, James high risk pregnancy, etc. (we cannot read the entire books again, atleast the important topics to be covered and highlight the important points for last minute revision).

But to refresh our MCQ tricks to crack the entrance exam you need to go back and read your entrance book read for NEET-PG preparation (we read Sakshi Arora Obstetrics and Gynaecology recent edition and 20-20 SERIES Reproductive endocrinology by Dr Aswath Kumar and Dr Nilesh Balkawade, it must be in your tips)

For Reproductive Endocrinology: *Leon Speroff* recent edition must be read (no other option) and do not forget to make your own notes/highlight important points for revision.

To get an idea about the pattern of questions you can refer online available reproductive medicine MCQ questions in NBE website.

History related to reproductive medicine/USG/X-ray/Picture-based questions/recent advances in reproductive medicine are expected questions.

And at the last few questions on statistics are usually asked. These are especially related to your thesis methodology, basic research methods, sampling aspects, types of study designs, etc.

Contents Taught in the Program

It is a comprehensive formal 3-year training program in all aspects of reproductive medicine and surgery designed to provide the candidate with every opportunity to gain adequate knowledge and proficiency in the principles of diagnosis and evidence-based management.

The program also stresses the importance of clinical and basic research relevant to the subspeciality.

CLINICAL ROTATION

1. *Reproductive Medicine (25 months):* OPD, history taking and evaluation, USG, other relevant investigations—SSG, HSG, hysteroscopy, laparoscopy
2. *Urology:* 1 month for andrology, male sexual dysfunction
3. *Andrology lab:* 1 month, semen analysis and interpretation
4. *Reproductive Endocrinology:* 2 months
5. *Fetal medicine and perinatology:* 1 month
6. *Clinical Psychology and sexology:* 1 month
7. *Embryology lab:* 4 months
8. *Outside IVF center:* 1 month.

SYLLABUS

- Basic and Applied Sciences
  - Basic Anatomy and physiology of male and female reproductive system
  - Applied Pharmacology, Biochemistry and Pathology of the male and female reproductive system
  - *Physiology:* Menstrual cycle/ovulation
  - *Endocrinology:* Relevant to human reproduction—hypothalamic-pituitary-ovarian hormones.
    - *Ovarian Hormones:* Structure, Biosynthesis, Function, Mechanism of Action, and knowledge of autocrine and paracrine hormones.
    - Endocrine disturbances affecting reproduction such as thyroid and adrenal function.

- Physiologic and Pathophysiologic Alterations of the Neuroendocrine Components of the Reproductive Axis
- Normal puberty and pubertal disorders.
- Polycystic ovary syndrome and other hyperandrogenic states
- Abnormal Uterine Bleeding
- Disorders of Sex Development
- Reproductive Immunology and Its Disorders
• *Ultrasonography* in reproductive medicine
• *Endoscopic surgery,* both Hysteroscopy and Laparoscopy
• Diagnosis and management of male and female infertility
    - Ovulation Induction
    - Monitoring of Ovulation
    - Intrauterine Insemination
    - Controlled Ovarian Stimulation
    - Assisted reproductive technology (ART)
• *Embryology:* Gametogenesis and fertilization
• *Genetics:* Nomenclature/basic principle/preimplantation genetic diagnosis
• *Laboratory equipment:* Handling and maintenance, record keeping, quality control and quality assurance
• *Andrology laboratory:* Semen analysis and sperm function tests
• *Infertility:* Broad outlines of causes of male and female infertility. Workup of male and female partner.
• *ART:* Evolution and different technologies
    - *Processing sperm for various procedures:* For intrauterine insemination, in vitro fertilization (IVF), intracytoplasmic sperm injection (ICSI) (Fig. 8.1)
    - Processing samples of testicular/epididymal sperms
    - Embryology laboratory

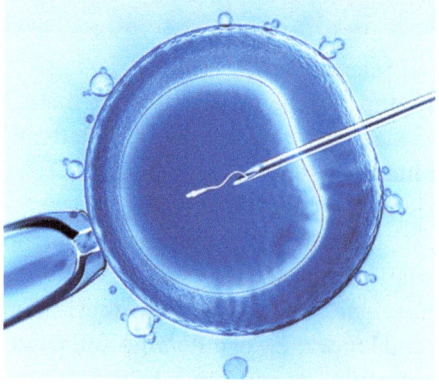

Fig. 8.1: Intracytoplasmic sperm injection (ICSI)

- Culture media
- Egg identification
- Insemination
- Normal/abnormal Fertilization and cleavage check.
- Blastocyst culture
- Embryo hatching
- Techniques of intracytoplasmic sperm injection
- Cryopreservation
- Principles of cryopreservation
- Semen freezing/oocyte freezing/ embryo freezing
- Slow freeze techniques/vitrification
- Ovum pick up and embryo transfer
- Safety issue in ART including ovarian hyperstimulation syndrome (OHSS) and multiple pregnancies
- Embryology lab quality control and maintenance
- Exposure to laboratory techniques in ART
- Storage and use of gametes
- Basics of reproductive genetics

- Genetic history and counseling
- Preimplantation genetic diagnosis
- Preimplantation genetic screening
- Endometrial Receptivity assay
- Ethical principles in ART.

After completion of the course, the reproductive medicine specialist will be proficient in the following areas of learning:

1. Operative gynecological open surgery, minimally invasive surgery and microsurgery.
2. Reproductive endocrinology and its management.
3. Proficient in the etiology, pathophysiology, diagnosis and management of common gynecological problems related to infertility like fibroids/endometriosis/pelvic infections/ectopic pregnancy and management of high order pregnancy.
4. Expertise in the use of ovulation inducing agents and hormonal control of the menstrual cycle and controlled ovarian stimulation.
5. Follicular recruitment and oocyte retrieval procedure.
6. Understand and be able to manage OHSS.
7. Transvaginal ultrasonography with particular reference to follicular monitoring and early pregnancy scanning.
8. *Andrology:* Semen analysis and semen preparation
9. *Laboratory Technology:* Familiarity with ART laboratory equipment, maintenance and trouble shooting.
10. Oocyte identification and grading, embryo grading, micromanipulation, cell culture, freezing techniques, etc.

11. Medicolegal and ethical aspect
    - Third Party Reproduction
        - Oocyte donation
        - Embryo donation
        - Sperm donation
        - Surrogacy
    - *Ethical and medicolegal aspects of infertility management:* ICMR guidelines
12. Miscellaneous
    - Biostatics and Data management.
    - Fertility preservation: Social and Oncofertility.
    - Monitoring and treatment of early pregnancy after ART treatment
    - Research Methodology
    - Medical statistics
    - Writing and presenting a paper.

Minimal hands on available in the course:
- Assist 10 Proximal cornual block
- Perform 5 Tubal recanalization procedures
- Minimally Invasive Assist 20 diagnostic laparoscopies
- Assist 20 operative laparoscopies
- Perform 10 diagnostic laparoscopies
- Perform 10 operative laparoscopies
- Andrology Assist 20 PESA, TESA, TESE of testis
- Perform 5 PESA, TESA, TESE testis
- IVF Assist 25 Oocyte retrieval
- Perform 10 Oocyte retrieval
- Laboratory Observe 20 semen analysis and 20 sperm preparation
- Perform 10 semen analysis and 10 sperm wash procedures
- Follow up 5 cases of IVF and 5 ICSI retrieval to embryo transfer (written records).

This is just a minimum and you might be getting to do more.

OPPORTUNITIES AFTER DOING THE COURSE

The field of reproductive medicine is in the late expansion phase and it will be becoming fully saturated in a decade or two. However many teaching institutions are coming up with superspeciality courses including government institutions. Those who are interested in academics and teaching can pursue their career in
1. Institutions with FNB program
2. Institutions with MCh Program (Private or public sector)
3. Any teaching institution under OBGYN department as a separate unit.

Other Opportunities

- You can start your own center as you will be fully equipped to do so on completion of the course
- You can work in corporate hospitals and establish your own unit there (there is always a high demand indeed)
- You can associate with giants in the field of reproductive medicine (they will be readily welcoming as no much MCh candidates are coming out every year).

If you want to earn more, the Middle East and other countries are always welcoming you. The availability of a valid MCI recognized MCh degree will be having high demand outside India even.

It might help you to work in the UK or US provided you obtain other background requirements to do so. And the most important fact is that a law might come in the future demanding that IVF centers need to be run by a person qualified enough (with a valid degree) only. This is because of so many malpractices seen in many small units. These things might come as a bill or law like the upcoming ART bill.

So, the course is clearly useful. The process of entry is somewhat difficult as the NEET examination needs intense preparation. However, it is not a Himalayan task and those who really work for it will get through.

The OBGYN is no more an end specialty as we once thought of. It is expanding in such a way that all the disease conditions or physiological aspects have separate books on its own. The whole thing cannot be taken as a simple sailing and it needs dedicated reading and effort to get through. Hope we will be able to see more number of seats in *MCh Reproductive Medicine and Surgery* including the public sector so that more and more people can pursue this golden course.

Fellowship in Reproductive Medicine and Surgery

Rohan Palshetkar, Jiteeka Thakkar

INTRODUCTION

As an MBBS student, one is always excited about the prospect of following a residency program. But throughout your medical college days as well as your residency program, you are never taught about the life post-PG.

The start of residency is one of the most exciting and strenuous times of a resident. Residency in the field of obstetrics and gynecology is one of the most strenuous residency programs that one has to go through. The sleepless nights, the rounds, the preoperative preparations, the surgeries itself and then postoperative monitoring makes it no less difficult for residents. At the start of the program it feels that we are almost done and once the residency program is over, I can begin my practice. However obstetrics and gynecology is a vast field. It encompasses various superspecialties which are not always covered in the residency program such as reproductive medicine, endoscopy, oncology, fetal medicine, etc.

So now that you have cleared your masters in obstetrics and gynecology, you have to look at the future and how to broaden your horizon. In this chapter, we will discuss about the various pros and cons of doing in vitro fertilization (IVF) fellowships/DNB/MCH after your residency program.

First and foremost, what is a fellowship? It is an academic opportunity for a gynecologist to work with a consultant in a field of their choice (in this case, IVF). Depending on the type of fellowship, the fellowship may be paid or unpaid and could last from a few days to a couple of years. MCh in *reproductive medicine* is another option but the duration is of 3 years. FNB in reproductive medicine is a slightly shorter option, but it is still 2 years long. One of the most important aspects of these programs is that the student gets valuable exposure, experience, guidance and mentorship under a senior consultant. These programs are also a great way to make connections with various colleagues and seniors in the field (Tables 9.1 to 9.4).

You must consider many factors when choosing one of these programs:
1. Am I interested in the field of IVF? Do I want to do IVF in the future?
2. How long do I want to do a program for?
3. Is this opportunity going to be my career?
4. Do I have what it takes to do one of these programs?

Table 9.1: List of Indian College of Obstetricians and Gynecology (ICOG) recognized centers for certificate course in reproductive medicine

S. No.	List of Centers	Courses available (6 months courses)
1.	Dr Mrs Shah Duru Sushil Kwality House, 1st Floor, Kemp's Corner, Mumbai 400 026. Tel: ® 2369 05 82. © 2380 25 84. Fax: 2380 48 39. E-mail: durushah@gmail.com Mobile: 9820074875	Reproductive Medicine.
2.	Dr Jaideep Malhotra Global Rainbow Healthcare, NH-2, Near Guru Ka Tal Gurudwara, Agra-7. Mobile : 09897033335 Tel: (0562)2260275/2260276/2260277/ 2260279 Fax: (0562)2265194. E-mail: jaideepmalhotraagra@gmail.com	Reproductive Medicine
3.	Dr Mrs. Shanti Roy V 19, Vidyapuri P.O., Lohianagar, Patna 800 020. Mobile: 9334105868, 9334105807 E-mail: Himanshu Roy (himanshuroy@hotmail.com), shantiroy40@gmail.com	Reproductive Medicine
4.	Dr Sanjay Anant Gupte Gupte Hospital, 894, Bhandarkar Road, Deccan Gymkhana, Poona 411 004. Tel: (9520) ® 2565 60 73. © 25653684/ 25661237. Fax: (9520) 2566 12 37. E-mail: guptehospital@gmail.com Mobile: 98220 30238	▪ Reproductive Medicine ▪ Ultrasound
5.	Dr Prakash Trivedi 501/502, Sai Heritage, Opp. Dr. Trivedi's Hospital, Above Axis Bank, Tilak Road, Ghatkopar East, Mumbai 400 077. Tel: © 515 88 75/515 89 20. Fax: 513 59 13/516 11 38. Mobile: 98200 52631.- out of station E-mail: dr.ptrivedi@gmail.com/ ptrivedi1702@gmail.com	▪ Reproductive Medicine ▪ Gynecological Endoscopy ▪ Ultrasonography
6.	Dr Sunita Tandulwadkar Grant Medical Foundation Ruby Hall Clinic, 40, Sasson Road, Pune-411001. Tel: 020-66455100 Mobile: 9822015850 E-mail: sunitart@hotmail.com, rubyhallivf@hotmail.com	▪ Reproductive Medicine ▪ Gynecological Endoscopy and Minimal Access Surgery

Contd...

Contd...

S. No.	List of Centers	Courses available (6 months courses)
7.	Dr Madhuri Patil Dr Patil's Fertility and Endoscopy clinic, 1, Uma Admiralty, First Floor, Bannerghatta Road, Bangalore-560029. Tel: 080-41201357/41462419 Mobile: 9945221622/9 E-mail: drmadhuripatil59@gmail.com	Reproductive Medicine
8.	Dr Padma Rekha Jirge 2013 E, 6th Lane, Rajarampuri, Kolhapur-416008 E-mail: saccivf@gmail.com Tel: 0231-2527765 Mobile: 09822114131	Reproductive Medicine
9.	Dr Jayam Kannan 8 C/D, Ramarayar Street, Tennur Trichy-620017, Tamil Nadu Tel: (0431) 4023201 ® 24844718 (O) Mobile: 09382828429 E-mail: triogstrichy@gmail.com Mobile: 09841795116 (Reena)	Reproductive Medicine
10.	Dr Vidya V Bhat Radhakrishna Multispeciality Hospital, 3-4, SUNRISE TOWERS JP Road, Girinagar Bangalore-560085 Tel: 080-26422977/88 Mobile: 9880128666/9448080319 E-mail: vidyabhat68@gmail.com	• Gynecological Endoscopy and Minimal Access Surgery • Reproductive Medicine
11.	Dr Ratna Thakur, Indore 144, Radio Colony, Indore 452010 Madhya Pradesh Tel: ® 2712626 © 49321000 Mobile: 9425056659 E-mail: ashokkumarthakur@gmail.com Pan Number: ABAPT7333C	• Reproductive Medicine • Gynecological • Endoscopy and Minimal Access Surgery • Ultrasonography
12.	Dr Parag Biniwale 942/4-B, Anupam Model Colony, Shivajinagar, Pune 411 016, Maharashtra Tel: ® (020)25671631 © 25656528 Mobile: 9822023061 Fax: (020) 24464181 E-mail: paragbin@vsnl.com/ parag.biniwale@gmail.com	• Reproductive Medicine

Contd...

Contd...

S. No.	List of Centers	Courses available (6 months courses)
13.	Dr Purnima Nadkarni 21st Century Hospital and Test Tube Baby Center, 51/B, Dawer Plaza, Sufi Baug, Near Savera Hotel, Station Road (Una Pani), Surat-395003 Gujarat Tel: 0261-2490190/2492190 Mobile: 09825135793 E-mail: nadkarnihospital@gmail.com, surat21st@rediffmail.com	• Reproductive Medicine
14.	Dr S Sankari Samundi Srushti Hospital Pvt. Ltd., Maternal and Child Health, Fertility and Multispeciality, No-1, Padmavathy Street Thirumalali Nagar, Ramapuram, Chennai-600089. Tel: 044-24861144, 24863544 M: 09840453454/09840039939 E-mail: sfrc@srushtihospital.com, drsssankari@yahoo.com	• Reproductive Medicine
15.	Dr S Krishnakumar JK Women Hospital, Maitri Raghukul, Shaheed Bhagat Singh Road, Opp. Saraswat Bank, Dombivali East-421201 Thane E-mail: rkjkrish@gmail.com Mobile: 9820067318/ Tel: (0251)2470797/2448693	• Gynecological Endoscopy • Reproductive Medicine
16.	Dr Asha Rao Rao Hospital, 120, West Periasamy Road, RS Puram, Coimbatore-641002 E-mail: asharao55@gmail.com raohospital2009@gmail.com Mobile: 09994354593/09003334329	• Reproductive Medicine • Gynecological Endoscopy
17.	Dr Sonia Malik Southend Fertility and IVF Center, 2, Palam Marg, Near Flyover, Vasant Vihar, New Delhi-110057 Tel: 011-26894767/26153635 Mobile: 09810122337 E-mail: sm_doc@hotmail.com sm_doc@southendivf.com	Reproductive Medicine
18.	Dr Bharati Dhorepatil Smile IVF Test Tube Center and Reproductive Medicine Unit, Shree Hospital, Siddharth Mansion, Nagar Road, Pune 411006 Tel: 022-26681127 Mobile: 09822043112 Ssmileivf@gmail.com	Reproductive Medicine

Contd...

Contd...

S. No.	List of Centers	Courses available (6 months courses)
19.	Dr Vasundra Thiagarajan New Life Fertility and IVF Center, BM Hospital, 36, 5th Main Road, Thillai Ganga Nagar, Nanganallur, Chennai-600061 Email: tpa@bmhospitals.com/ dr.vasundra@bmhospitals.com Mobile: 9841061182	Reproductive Medicine
20.	Dr Nutan Jain Vardhman Trauma and Laparoscopy Center Pvt. Ltd., Vardhman Test Tube Center, 36, South Civil Line, Mahaveer Chowk, Muzaffarnagar-251001 UP. Mobile: 08393008866/09720675029 E-mail: jainnutan@gmail.com/ vandanamamac03@gmail.com	Reproductive Medicine
21.	Dr Chaitanya Shembekar Shembekar Hospital Pvt. Ltd., OMEGA Hospital, 53, LIC Colony, Khamla Road, Near Ajni Square, Nagpur-440015 Mobile: 0 9822572744 E-mail: chaitanyashembekar@yahoo.com	Reproductive Medicine

Table 9.2: List of DM (Reproductive Medicine)/MCh (Reproductive Medicine and Surgery) (MCI website)

S. No.	Medical College	No of Seats
1	Sri Aurobindo Medical College and Post Graduate Institute, Indore	2
2	Sri Ramachandra Medical College and Research Institute, Chennai	2

Table 9.3: List of FNB centers for reproductive medicine.

S. No.	Center	No of Seats
1.	Sir Gangaram Hospital, Delhi	2
2.	Lok Nayak Jai Prakash (LNJP) Hospital, Delhi	2
3.	Nova Pulse IVF Clinic, Ahmedabad	1
4.	Bangalore Assisted Conception Center (BACC), Bengaluru	4
5.	Bangalore Baptist Hospital, Bangalore	1
6.	Craft Hospital and Research Center, Trichur	1
7.	Ruby Hall Clinic, Pune	2
8.	Lilavati Hospital and Research Center, Mumbai	1
9.	Madras Medical Mission Hospital, Chennai	2
10.	Oasis Center for Reproductive Medicine, Hyderabad	2

Table 9.4: List of university recognized fellowship.

S. No.	University	Duration
1.	Dr DY Patil University, Navi Mumbai	1 year
2.	Rajiv Gandhi University of Health Sciences	1 and half years
3.	Manipal University	1 year
4.	The Tamil Nadu Dr MGR Medical University	2 years

ARE YOU INTERESTED IN THE FIELD OF IVF? DO I WANT TO DO IVF IN THE FUTURE?

As a resident, you may not be sure about the field of superspecialty you want to choose. If you are not sure about the field, then it is ideal to take a fellowship program of a shorter duration as you will get an idea about the field. You as a fellow are exposed to the latest technology available. Therefore when you have done the fellowship, you know all the available treatments that you can provide to your patients in the future. Another advantage is that many of the fellowships available in India provide hands on training to the fellows. Therefore as a part of the fellowship, you will learn various procedures for the first time, which you probably have not been exposed to in residency. However, the hands on procedures will probably be available only if you pursue a longer course. When you are in a longer duration fellowship, you develop a bond with your mentor. This bond results into trust and your mentor will reward you with procedures. However with short-term fellowships, there is more of a chance that you will end up observing more than actually doing hands on procedures. However if you are sure about pursuing IVF as a career, then all three options are viable for you. MCh or FNB in reproductive medicine would be highly beneficial in the long-term, as they are recognized degrees and in addition, over these long-term periods, you would get a lot more hands on.

How Long do I want do a Program for?

As I already mentioned before, MCH program lasts for 3 years, while a FNB program is for 2 years. Fellowships can last from 1 month to as long as even 2 years in some places. So depending on how much time you are willing to commit for your training comes into play. It is of my opinion that you require a minimum of 6 months to 1 year to actually get a grasp of the field and also learn the tips and tricks from your mentor. It is not only the standard protocols you need to pay attention to but also small adjustment your mentor makes in order to make your practice easier.

Do I have What it Takes to do One of These Programs?

Firstly, there is no substitute to hard work. It all begins with the application forms. In order to enter MCh or FNB program, one needs to go through the preparation for vigorous entrance exams. Fellowship programs may or may not have entrance exams. Also during these programs, you need to put in the hard work you did during residency. Even after you finish the various duration of training, there is an exit exam for MCh, FNB and some fellowship programs as well.

What is Taught in These Programs?

These programs are self-explanatory. You will be given in-depth knowledge into the field of IVF. Courses will cover ultrasonography, laboratory set up as well as workings in the lab. You will be taught about evaluating an infertile couple and the counseling. Besides that you will be taught about the ethics involved in IVF which I believe is one of the most important concerns.

WHAT ARE THE OPPORTUNITIES AVAILABLE POST THESE FELLOWSHIPS?

The opportunities are immense post fellowships. There are multiple IVF centers which are looking for doctors in the field of reproductive medicine and with the help of your fellowship, you will be one step ahead than the others for job opportunities. Another option is that with all the knowledge you gain not only in the field of IVF but also in the setup of one, you can easily set up your own IVF center. It all depends on what your long-term goal is!

CHAPTER 10

Urogynecology Fellowship

Tanvir, Ajay Rane

INTRODUCTION

If you are reading this chapter, you may be considering applying for training in urogynecology. Obstetrics and gynecology (OBGYN) is a great mixture of medicine and surgery, often exciting, but also challenging. After specializing in OBGYN, you could train further to be a subspecialist in urogynecology. Although there is no formal training course for urogynecology in India, there are various ways to gain more experience in this highly specialized field and create a niche for yourself. It is often challenging for young specialists to find an overseas fellowship program, but not impossible. The aim of this chapter is to give you a glimpse of what really is involved. Training for urogynecology can vary from observership, hands on training to a fellowship.

WHO IS A UROGYNECOLOGIST?

Subspecialists in urogynecology or female pelvic medicine and reconstructive pelvic surgery (FPM-RPS) are defined as surgical clinicians, either obstetricians/gynecologists or urologists or colorectal surgeons, who provide comprehensive management to women with complex benign pelvic conditions, lower urinary tract disorders, and pelvic floor dysfunction.

Comprehensive management includes those diagnostic and therapeutic procedures necessary for the total care of the patient with these conditions and complications resulting from them.[1]

Most successful urogynecology units include multidisciplinary team of specialist nurses, physiotherapists, neurophysicians, trainee doctors and urogynecologists.[2]

Subspecialists in Urogynecology/FPM-RPS[1]

- Demonstrate detailed knowledge of the anatomy and physiology of the pelvis, the contained viscera and the pathological processes affecting their function.
- Clinical competence in the investigation and treatment of the disorders of function of the lower urinary tract in women, pelvic floor and anorectal function.

- They are in a position to establish and maintain a urogynecology/FPM-RPS unit and provide a referral service for women with complicated urinary and pelvic floor problems.
- They are active in research and teaching and concerned with the management of women with intractable urinary and/or fecal incontinence, and persistent pelvic floor dysfunction.

WHAT ARE THE GUIDELINES FOR TRAINING IN UROGYNECOLOGY?

International Urogynecological Association (IUGA) is the leading organization in this field and has established guidelines that are universally acceptable to various boards and colleges from around the world: Royal College of Obstetricians and Gynaecologists (RCOG), German Society of Urogynecology, Society of Obstetricians and Gynaecologists of Canada (SOGC), American Board of Obstetrics and Gynecology (ABOG), Royal Australian College of Obstetricians and Gynaecologists (RANZCOG), European Urogynecological Association (EUGA).[1,3]

Objectives for Subspecialization

- To improve the quality of care of women with pelvic floor disorders.
- To improve knowledge, practice, teaching and research in female pelvic health.
- To promote the concentration of specialized expertise, special facilities and clinical material that will be of considerable benefit to patients with female pelvic disorders and hence improve the quality of their care.
- To establish a close understanding and working relationship with other disciplines involved in the field of urogynecology/FPM-RPS.
- To encourage coordinated management of relevant clinical services throughout a region.
- To accept a major regional responsibility for higher training, research and audit in the subspecialty fields.
- Fellowship recognized programs should be expected to promote evidence-based medicine prior to the widespread clinical application of industry-driven new technology.

These objectives may vary from country to country.

Requirements for Trainees

In order to start subspecialization in Urogynecology/FPM-RPS the following requirements are mandatory:
- Trainees should be qualified physicians, certified by their national board as having successfully completed general residency training in obstetrics and gynecology or urology.

- The minimum requirements for entry into the clinical subspecialty of Urogynecology/FPM-RPS are dependent on national laws and regulations.
- The minimal requirement may vary from country to country.
- The minimum requirements for recognition as a subspecialist in Urogynecology/FPM-RPS are dependent on national laws and regulations, which may include board examination and certification.
- In order to register as a subspecialist in Urogynecology/FPM-RPS, the trainee should be able to demonstrate his or her skills by means of a list of performed diagnostic and therapeutic procedures, scientific publications and have the approval of the director of the training program to be recognized as subspecialist.[1,3]

WHAT ARE THE MINIMAL REQUIREMENTS TO PRACTICE UROGYNECOLOGY?

Several countries in the world may not have the resources, facilities, trained support staff or trained subspecialty physician capable of offering a subspecialty training in urogynecology. The FIGO Task Force has guidelines for resident/general physician training in offering minimal standards for urogynecology services for women. The requirements are listed below:[4]

Knowledge (knows both specifically and broadly) should include at least the following topics:
- Trauma and congenital anomalies that result in incontinence.
- Voiding dysfunction and urinary retention.
- Urinary incontinence types an assessment.
- Overactive bladder syndrome.
- Painful bladder syndrome/interstitial cystitis.
- Urinary tract infection.
- Lower urinary and intestinal tract fistulae.
- Pelvic pain syndrome.
- Pelvic organ prolapse.
- Childbirth related pelvic floor trauma.
- Urethral lesions, i.e. diverticula.
- Effects of surgery and irradiation on the lower urinary and intestinal tracts and pelvic floor function.
- Urinary disorders in pregnancy (including infections and incontinence).
- Evaluation and care of the elderly with pelvic floor disorders.
- Lesions of the central nervous system affecting urinary and feral control and pelvic floor function.
- Disorders of the lower intestinal tract including difficult defecation, fecal incontinence, and rectal prolapse.
- Obstetric anal sphincter injury.
- Emotional and behavioral disorders affecting the pelvic floor and lower urinary and intestinal tract function.
- Urinary disorders of childhood.

- Pelvic floor disorders in the physically and mentally challenged individual.
- Sexually transmitted diseases.
- Effect of hormone deficiency states on the pelvic floor.
- Urinary problems secondary to medical conditions and drugs.
- Sexual dysfunction and coital incontinence.
- Vulvar disorders.
- Principles of evidence-based medicine, epidemiology, and critical appraisal of urogynecologic research.
- Electronic and nonelectronic urodynamics studies.

Clinical competence (can be performed alone but may need assistance) should be acquired in at least the following skills by the end of training:

1. Take a urogynecologic history.
2. Perform a basic urogynecologic physical examination including neurologic and pelvic floor assessment.
3. Interpret urodynamic studies.
4. Assess and perform nonsurgical management of pelvic organ prolapse.
5. Treat acute bladder voiding disorders.
6. Counsel and plan initial management of overactive bladder, interstitial cystitis, stress urinary incontinence, and pelvic pain syndrome.
7. Perform the following operative procedures under direct supervision:
    a. Primary repair of anterior and posterior vaginal prolapse.
    b. Vaginal hysterectomy
    c. Enterocele repair
    d. Suburethral sling procedure
8. Observe and/or assist in the following procedures:
    a. Diagnostic cystourethroscopy, particularly to rule out cystotomy, intravesical or intraurethral suture or mesh placement, and to verify bilateral ureteral patency during or after gynecological surgical procedures.
    b. Colposuspension procedure.
    c. Complex vaginal vault suspensions.
    d. Repair of rectovaginal fistula anal sphincteroplasty.
    e. Cystoscopy and periurethral injection.

The subspeciality training programs in urogynecology are not available in India as of 2018.

There are three societies that offering are:

1. Urogynecology Committee of FOGSI.
2. URPSSI—Urogynecology and Reconstructive Pelvic Surgery Society of India in association with IUGA.
3. UPIA—Urogynecology Pelvic Floor Dysfunction and Incontinence Association.

Every year Dr Vineet Mishra, Head of the Department and Professor of Obstetrics and Gynecology, Institute of Kidney Diseases and Research Center, Institute of Transplantation Sciences, Ahmedabad, Gujarat holds yearly an urogynecology congress in December.

What is the Length of Training and Registration as Subspecialist in Urogynecology/FPM-RPS?

Observership
Duration: 2 weeks to 6 months

Fellowship
Duration: 1-2 Years

Certification Course
Duration: 3 Years

Trainees should be qualified and certified by their national board.

What You Can Learn From an Observership?

- Observership duration range from 2 weeks to 6 months.
- Have an aim and be very specific about what you want to learn.
- It would be a good beginning for young aspiring urogynecologists.

The curriculum consists of:

- *Attending the clinics:* Observe history taking, clinical examination, translabial/transperineal pelvic floor ultrasound (including 3D/4D), endoanal ultrasonography (3D/4D), anorectal manometry, and complete pelvic floor neurophysiologic testing. Discussion of the cases with the experts.
- *Attending the Urodynamic study:* Observe and learn how the machine is arranged, interpretation of its findings, and its influence on the management.
- Attend operation theater and observe various procedures such as TVT, TVT-O, Botox, prolapse surgeries with or without mesh, laparoscopic sacrocolpopexy, fistula repair, and many more.
- Observers in some units may have opportunities to work on small research projects.

IUGA provides observational grants and details of which can be accessed from the *www.iuga.org*. Once you click on this, go into the grant section to find details.

What You Can Learn From Fellowship?

The fellowship duration ranges from 1 year to 3 years. The trainee must demonstrate a thorough knowledge of anatomy, physiology and pharmacology of the lower urinary tract and the impact of pregnancy, parturition, menopause and aging on lower urinary tract system.

Conditions to be familiar with:

- Urodynamic stress incontinence
- Detrusor overactivity
- Trauma and congenital abnormalities resulting in incontinence
- Voiding disorders and urinary retention
- Overactive bladder syndrome

- Pelvic pain
- Lower urinary tract and lower gastrointestinal tract fistulae
- Pelvic organ prolapse, both primary and recurrent
- Painful bladder syndrome
- Urethral lesions, e.g. diverticula
- Effects of pelvic surgery and irradiation on the lower bowel urinary tract and pelvic floor
- Urinary disorders in pregnancy
- Evaluation and care of the elderly
- Lesions of the central nervous system affecting urinary, fecal control and pelvic floor
- Difficult defection
- Disorders of lower gastrointestinal tract function including incontinence and motility
- Obstetric anal sphincter injury (OASIS)
- Urinary disorders in childhood
- The physically or mentally handicapped
- Sexually transmitted diseases
- Emotional and behavioral disorders
- Hormone deficiency states
- Urinary problems secondary to medical disorders and drugs
- Symptoms associated with sexual intercourse, e.g. coital incontinence.

History

Learning Objectives

- To demonstrate the knowledge skills and attitudes required to make an appropriate clinical assessment of an urogynecological patient.
- To understand the different facets of obtaining a history of the woman's condition:
    - Obtain a general history
    - Obtain a urinary/prolapse/bowel and sexual history
    - Use standardized questionnaires
    - Use quality of life questionnaire

Examination

Learning Outcomes

- To be able to carry out a competent examination:
    - Undertake a general examination
    - Undertake a pelvic examination, including standardized methods of assessment
    - Undertake a relevant neurological examination

Investigation

Learning Outcomes

- To be able to select appropriate tests and carry out the test proficiently and where appropriate interpret results.

Conservative Management of Urogynecological Condition

Learning Outcomes

- To demonstrate a thorough understanding of the evaluation and treatment of lower urinary tract disorders using conservative measures (including recommendations of the International Consultation on Incontinence)
  - Anatomy and function of lower urinary tract and pelvis
  - Fluid management
  - Physical therapies
  - Pharmacological therapies
  - Catheters and drug therapies for voiding difficulties
  - Pessaries for prolapse
  - Other therapies.

Surgical Outcomes

Learning Outcomes

- To demonstrate the knowledge and skills to understand the indications for and the ability to carry out the required surgical procedures. This includes the skills and attitudes to counsel patients appropriately, to have an understanding of potential surgical complications, failure rates and how to deal with them when they occur.

Neurology

Learning Outcomes

- To understand the effects of neurological conditions on the lower urinary tract
- To understand and have knowledge of the principles of specialist assessment and treatments for bladder dysfunction.

Laparoscopic Urogynecology

Learning Outcomes

- To be able to select patients who are suitable to be offered laparoscopic urogynecology
- To have a thorough knowledge of the equipment and resources required to deliver safe laparoscopic surgical care including different energy sources

- To be able to counsel patients on the benefits, risks and complications of laparoscopic procedures and obtain consent
- To observe and assist laparoscopic sacrocolpopexy and sacrohysteropexy
- To have the opportunity to observe other laparoscopic urogynecology procedures
- To understand regional referral pathways for complex and recurrent cases.[5]

Which Centers Provide Fellowship and Observership?

- Check the list on www.iuga.org: IUGA Fellowship and Observership Host Site Directory.
- Professor Ajay Rane, Urogynaecology Unit, Mater Misericordiae Hospital, Queensland, Australia.
    - *Click on the link for details:* http://www.femalepelvichealth.com.au/courses_training.html
    - They offer the 4 weeks and 12 weeks course, most suitable for specialists to get an overview of the speciality.
    - *1-year fellowship*
- Asia pacific urogynecology Association offers International fellowship programme for trainees in Asia-Pacific area.
    - *Click on the link for details:* http://www.apuga.org/education/Training.asp
    - 1–3 years fellowship
- Short courses are offered by International Academy of Pelvic Surgery.
    - *Program Directors:* Dr Mickey Karram and Dr Mark D Walters.
    - *Click on the link for details:* https://academyofpelvicsurgery.com

Kindly check the above websites for details regarding the visa application and other requirements of each country. Some countries take as long as 3–4 months for processing the application. Best approach is to contact the unit to express your interest.

Am I Eligible to do a Certificate Course in Urogynecology with an Indian MS/MD Degree in OBGYN?

No.

If I want to Take up MS/MD OBGYN and Specialize in Urogynecology Post-MBBS, How Do I Proceed?

As already said, there are no urogynecology programs available in India as of 2018. Few questions you need to answer is:
- Would you settle in India or overseas?
- Would you study OBGYN in India or overseas?
- Do you want to do exclusive urogynecology work?

WHAT ARE THE OPPORTUNITIES AFTER UROGYNECOLOGY FELLOWSHIP IN INDIA?

Exclusive urogynecology is been practiced by very few physicians. The ideal practice is multidisciplinary team work. The medical system of practice in India is not strictly referral base. Single clinical urogynecological units take time to get recognized.

Unfortunately, due to lack of awareness, issues of prolapse and incontinence are treated as normal part of aging. Many women suffer in silence and have poor quality of life. As a specialist with further training in urogynecology there are great opportunities in India. Pioneering healthcare in pelvic function would be extremely satisfying and improving quality of life for many such women is essential.

I would like to end by quoting Dr Peter L Dywer "Finally, the acquisition of knowledge and wisdom never stops. I find I learn new things every day, not only from my colleagues and fellows, but also from my patients. They have taught me to be conservative in my treatment whenever possible, to try to do more good than harm, and that why you are operating is just as important as how you operate."[6]

ACKNOWLEDGMENT

I would like to express my special thanks to Dr Meeta and Dr Mugdha Kulkarni for their assistance in reviewing this manuscript.

REFERENCES

1. IUGA Educational Committee. Urogynecology and Reconstructive. Pelvic Surgery. Int Urogynecol J. 2002;13:386.
2. Smith AR. Teaching and learning in urogynecology. Int Urogynecol J. 2014;25:15.
3. IUGA Training Site Directory. Int Urogynecol J (2016) 27: 325. https://doi.org/10.1007/s00192-015-2937-9.
4. Stenchever MA, et al. Int J Gynecol Obstet. 2007;107:187-90.
5. RCOG. Urogynaecology curriculum. London: RCOG; 2018.
6. Peter L. Dwyer. My mentors in urogynecology. International Urogynecology Journal. 2016;27(12):1783-4.

CHAPTER 11

Public Health Sector and Family Planning

Varsha Dange

INTRODUCTION

In a developing country like India, the maternal mortality ratio is still a great concern! Working in community or social medicine creates a realization in the gynecological surgeons about the impacts toward the country and humanity through his/her health service delivery.

Government jobs imparting health service delivery in public health sector are gaining popularity in Modern India! This is due to its vastly available alluring opportunities across the country. The public health sector working for maternal and child health contributes huge efforts in reducing maternal morbidity and mortality in India and internationally too. A Gynecologist and an Obstetrician can associate with Community Medicine by rendering his/her services through working with Central, State, District and Local self-Government agencies, ESIC hospitals, National and International Non-governmental organizations (NGOs), medical colleges, Indian defense/railway services all over India. The services can be on a full time, part time, consultancy or adhoc basis.

INDIAN SCENARIO

Opportunities with Central Government of India

The Government of India provides various vacancies in medical field on different platforms, to name a few, Ministry of Health And Family Welfare,[1] Medical Colleges as AIIMS, PGIMER, JIPMER, NIMHANS, etc. Railway Hospitals, Defense services (Short Service and Permanent commissions) also through Union Public Service Commission![2] All the opportunities and details are advertised on these organization's official websites as well as in leading newspapers and on websites such as *devnetjobsIndia.org*.[3] Usual way of selection is either written tests or interview or both may be resorted by these organizations for recruitment. There are reservation norms for all the posts. The pay scale for these posts is according to the pay commissions in force at the time of appointment. The pay scales may differ as per the institution and the hierarchy of the post. At present, the pay scale is according to 6th/7th pay commission[4-7] recommendations in pay band 15,600–39,100 with differing grade pays as 5,400, 6,600, etc. summing up in a decent take home salary. The Indian government revises the salaries for its employees according to the pay commission's recommendations on time-to-time basis. Also after completing tenure of service, one is entitled for pension according to the pension scheme[8] in force at the time of joining the service.

Union Public Service Commission (UPSC) helps various central government agencies, e.g. Railways, Indian Ordnance Factories, Delhi Municipal Corporation, Central Health Services, etc. for recruitment of medical officers (MO) or specialists by implementing the selection process. UPSC invites online applications and conducts nationwide examination for this. The examination consists of multiple choice questionnaires on medical subjects with negative marking system. The centers for examinations are placed all over India.

Medical Teaching

Another lucrative field is being a teacher to shape up budding doctors. For teaching an undergraduate or a postgraduate medical student, first we need to acquire qualifications laid down in act by Medical Council of India (MCI) in gazette "Minimum Qualifications for Teachers in Medical Institutions Regulations, 1998" (amended up to June 8th, 2017).[9]

According to these regulations Medical Teachers in all Medical Colleges except the Tutors, Residents, Registrars and Demonstrators must possess the requisite recognized postgraduate medical qualification in their respective subject. For the teachers who want to work as Assistant Professor, Associate Professor and Professor, the eligibility criteria are given in Table 11.1.

Senior Resident (Broad Specialties)

A *senior resident* is one who is doing his/her residency in the concerned postgraduate subject after obtaining PG degree (MD/MS) and is less than 40 years of age.

As per these regulations, a fresher who has just acquired postgraduation degree has to join senior residency to pursue his/her career in teaching in Broad Specialties. The qualifications required for teaching superspecialties are in accordance with the Table 11.1, the experience is considered after acquiring a superspecialty degree.

The pay scale of medical teachers is in accordance with University Grants Commission.[10] The basic pay band is same as described earlier for 6/7th pay commission recommendations but the grade pay is way higher for medical teachers. Another greater advantage is the age of retirement. One can remain the teaching faculty up to 65–70 years of age.

Table 11.1: Minimum qualifications for teachers in medical institutions as per Medical Council of India (MCI).

Posts	Qualification requirement	Teaching and research experience
Assistant Professor	A postgraduate qualification (PG) MD/MS in the concerned subject and as per the Teachers' Eligibility Qualifications (TEQ) Regulations	3 years Junior Resident in a recognized medical college in the concerned subject and 1 year as Senior Resident in the concerned subject in a recognized medical college
Associate Professor (5-year Post-PG experience)	A PG qualification MD/MS in the concerned subject and as per TEQ Regulation	As Assistant Professor in the subject for 4 years in a permitted/approved/recognized medical college/institution with 2 Research Publication in Indexed Journals as first Author or as corresponding author
Professor/Additional Professor (8-year of Post-PG experience)	A PG qualification MD/MS in the concerned subject and as per the TEQ Regulations	Associate Professor in the subject for 3 years in a permitted/approved/recognized medical college/institution with 4 Research Publications in Indexed Journal on Cumulative basis with minimum of 2 Research Publication during the tenure of Associate Professor as first Author or as corresponding author

State Government Avenues

Each state government has its own public health departments (PHD)[11] throughout India. The state government appoints all the specialists through its own public health department or its public service commissions. These posts are advertised on the official websites of PHD or Public Service Commissions' websites as well as in the leading newspapers. The written tests followed by interviews are the usual course for the selection and appointment. The reservation norms are followed during the recruitment process. After the appointment, one can start working in capacity of a MO Class 2 or may directly join as a class 1 Gynecologist. These MOs/Specialists may be placed in any of the PHC/Rural/Sub-district/District/Women's hospitals throughout the State, on a full time basis. The pay scale for these posts is according to the pay commissions in force at the time of appointment. At present, the pay scale is according to 6th pay commission recommendations, e.g. for a class one officer the payment is in 15,600–39,100 grade pay 6,600 amounting to gross salary of INR 72,000 and class 2 MO is 15,600–39,100 grade pay 5,400 with gross salary of INR 68,000. The Indian government revises the salary according to the pay commission's recommendations.

The State Government of Maharashtra awards, Class 2 MOs and Specialists, additional 6 increments for achieved postgraduate degree and 3 additional increments[12] for achieved postgraduate diploma qualifications along with routine salary.

Maharashtra Public Service Commission (MPSC) conducts examinations for the selection of MOs/Specialists for PhD, Maharashtra in the similar manner as done by UPSC. Many times intradepartmental promotion process of specialists or medical officers for PhD is also conducted by MPSC.

The *National Health Mission* (NHM) has opened new boulevard in employments of specialists.[13] Under NHM, specialists are recruited in FRUs/RH/SDH by districts. The Specialist posts are advertised at district level through District Civil Surgeon. The contractual gynecologist under NHM will be offered remuneration as shown in Table 11.2.

Municipal Corporations

The municipal corporations, municipal councils are the independent local bodies with its own health system administered separately from district and state government. Corporations/Councils follow the similar process of recruitment as state government to appoint specialists/MOs. Pay scales are as per 6th pay commission and at par with state government. Working with corporations provides a great opportunity of staying in urban place.

Working with Nongovernmental Organizations in India

Many nongovernmental organizations (NGOs) nowadays work in the field of maternal and child health. The projects contribute in reducing maternal morbidity and mortality through working in areas like adolescent health, safe abortion services, antenatal and postpartum care, contraceptive practices, gynecological cancers, etc. One can be associated with them as a clinical mentor, program manager, researcher, freelance consultant. This can be on a part-time or a full time basis. The work profile may range from training the HR, collecting, organizing, recording and analyzing the data and performing research, advocacy on different levels, and program management along with actual clinical work. Few NGOs working in India through their nationwide projects are IPAS for Comprehensive Abortion Care, JHEPIEGO in Advanced Family Planning, ENGENDER HEALTH, ACCESS, SNEHA—all in maternal and child health and family planning. Also UNFPA, USAID still remain the major NGOs working internationally. All the career options are majorly advertised on these organizations websites. All these job profiles most of the times need additional masters' qualifications in public health. Various universities/institutes in India offer Masters in Public Health (MPH) which are Public Health Foundation of India—New Delhi, Gandhi Nagar, Bhubaneswar, Hyderabad; Tata Institute of Social Sciences, Mumbai; Indian

Table 11.2: Specialist cadre remuneration [Obstetrician/Gynecologist (OB/GYN)].

Name of Post	Type of appointment	Remuneration per month (In ₹)			Terms and condition of remuneration	Duty and job responsibility
		Non-TSP Blocks	Coastal District	TSP Block		
OBGYN	Full time Fixed monthly amount (In ₹) (a)	50,000	60,000	70,000	1. In order to get fixed monthly amount, it is mandatory to operate minimum 5 LSCS in a month. 2. In case of 5 or more than 5 LSCS operation in a month, the Gynecologist will receive both amounts (a+b) with excluding OPD charges, i.e. Fixed monthly amount as well as performance based amount as mentioned in visits basis/on call basis criteria. 3. In case of less than 5 LSCS, i.e. between 0 and 4 LSCS in a month, then Gynecologist will not get fixed monthly amount (a). However, Gynecologist will receive only performance-based amount (b) as mentioned in visit basis/on call basis criteria. Total monthly salary = b only	OPD from 9.00 am to 1.00 pm and 4.00 pm to 6.00 pm 6 days a week +IPD (including post-operative care) 2 rounds per day for 7 days a week + emergency calls
	On call basis/event basis performance based amount (in ₹) (b)				• LSCS procedure (with postoperative care) ₹ 4,000 per case for Non-TSP Blocks, Coastal District • LSCS procedure (with postoperative care) ₹ 6,000 per case for TSP Blocks • OPD/ANC/PNC checkup ₹ 50/case (maximum allowable limit ₹ 2,000 per day). • Assist in delivery ₹ 1,500/case • Other major surgery ₹ 4,000 per case (with postoperative care) • Other minor surgery ₹ 2,000 per case (with postoperative care). Other terms and conditions—no TA/DA will be given for on call/visit	On call criteria for LSCS and ANC/PNC as per laid down by RCH Programme

Institute of Health Management and Research, Jaipur; Institute of Public Health, Bengaluru; Savitribai Phule University, Pune; Maharashtra University of Health Sciences, Nasik; KLE University, Belgaum. MPH is a fulltime 2-year Masters' degree course. Acquiring this may help while working in Public Health and Family Medicine on International Platform too.

Family Planning

India is the first country to implement any sort of Family Planning program. In all Medical Colleges across India, separate Family Planning Department is run under a dedicated consultant—Assistant or Associate Professor or similar cadre. Also the district hospitals/Women's Hospitals have a dedicated wing working for sexual health and family planning requiring Gynecologist services.

There are few NGOs who exclusively work for sexual health and family planning, e.g. Family Planning Association of India (FPAI)[14] offers courses in laparoscopic female sterilization for DGO and MS (OBGYN) graduates.

THE INTERNATIONAL HORIZON

Working for maternal health and family planning has a huge scope on international platform.

There are fellowships and masters' degree programs in family planning and family medicine in many universities across the globe, e.g. in United States, fully funded 2-year fellowships in Family Planning[15] are offered in 30 universities.

Each country has its own entrance examinations to enter their medical education system, added to our baseline education earned in India.

The duration of these fellowship program ranges from few months up to 2 years. After completing the Masters or fellowships, one can work with NGOs or Hospitals as a consultant in Family Planning or Family Medicine. Even WHO and other international agencies as UNAIDS, UNFPA, etc. prefers these graduates.

REFERENCES

1. Ministry of Health and Family Welfare, India. [online] Available from https://mohfw.gov.in/. [Accessed November, 2018].
2. Union Public Service Commission. [online] Available from http://www.upsc.gov.in/. [Accessed November, 2018].
3. DevNetJobsIndia. [online] Available from http://www.devnetjobsindia.org/. [Accessed November, 2018].
4. Central Pay Commission, Ministry of Expenditure. CPC decision. [online] Available from https://doe.gov.in/sites/default/files/6cpcdecision%20%281%29.pdf. [Accessed November, 2018].

5. Central Pay Commission, Ministry of Expenditure. Pay notification. [online] Available from https://www.nitt.edu/home/righttoinfoact/6th_payNotification.pdf. [Accessed November, 2018].
6. Central Pay Commission, Ministry of Expenditure, 7th CPC resolution. [online] Available from https://www.finmin.nic.in/sites/default/files/7thCPC_resolution25072016.pdf? download=1. [Accessed November, 2018].
7. Central Pay Commission, Ministry of Expenditure, 7 CPC. [online] Available from https://www.finmin.nic.in/seven-cpc. [Accessed November, 2018].
8. Pensioners Portal. New Pension Scheme. [online] Available from http://pensionersportal.gov.in/salient%20features-f.asp. [Accessed November, 2018].
9. Medical Council of India. Minimum Qualifications for Teachers in Medical Institutions Regulations, 1998 (Amended upto 8th June, 2017). [online] Available from https://www.mciindia.org/documents/rulesAndRegulations/Teachers-Eligibility-Qualifications-Rgulations-1998.pdf. [Accessed November, 2018].
10. University grants Commission. Revision of Pay of teachers. [online] Available from https://www.ugc.ac.in/pdfnews/7077481_Revision-of-Pay-of-teachers.pdf. [Accessed November, 2018].
11. Public Health Department, Government of Maharashtra. [online] Available fromhttps://arogya.maharashtra.gov.in. [Accessed November, 2018].
12. State Government of Maharashtra. Government Resolutions (GR No. 20111214095222001/GR No. 201211191419253917). [online] Available from https://www.maharashtra.gov.in/Site/Common/governmentResolutions.aspx. [Accessed November, 2018].
13. National Health Mission. NHM/Specialists Guidelines. [online] Available from https://mohfw.gov.in/sites/default/files/. [Accessed November, 2018].
14. Family Planning Association of India. [online] Available from http://www.fpaindia.org/. [Accessed November, 2018].
15. Fellowships in Family Planning. [online] Available from https://www.familyplanningfellowship.org/. [Accessed November, 2018].

CHAPTER 12

MRCOG: A Roadmap

Megha Jayprakash

INTRODUCTION

I have compiled the information given on various sections on the RCOG website as well as added tips of my own and of some who have passed the exam recently. The idea of writing such a chapter was to make the long and sometimes challenging journey toward the coveted membership easier for the Membership of Royal College of Obstetricians and Gynaecologists (MRCOG) aspirant.

OVERVIEW OF THE UK SYSTEM OF TRAINING

The Royal College of Obstetricians and Gynaecologists sets the standards for the structure of training and the curriculum which is approved by the General Medical Council (GMC) (Fig. 12.1). Once this training program is completed, Certificate of Completion of Training (CCT) is awarded. This is required for entry onto the Specialist Register.

All UK trainees entering specialty training need to subscribe to the RCOG Trainees Register to receive their ePortfolio (eLogbook included) and other benefits. They will receive a unique National Training Number (NTN).

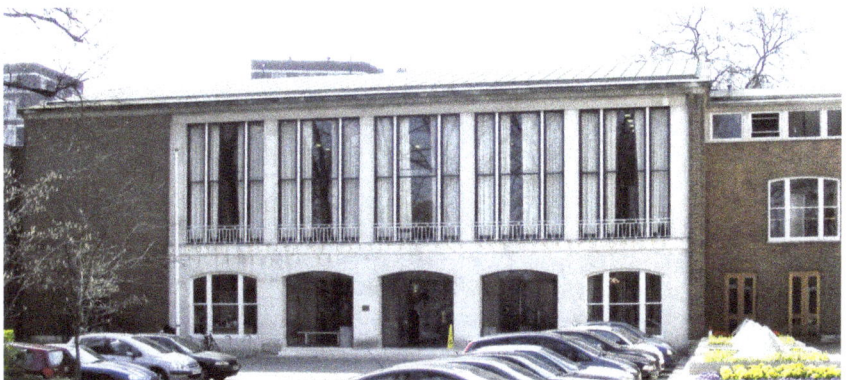

Fig. 12.1: Royal College of Obstetricians and Gynaecologists headquarters in London.

The specialty training curriculum in obstetrics and gynaecology (O&G) is competency-based and most trainees starting at ST-1 will take 7 years to reach ST-7 and complete their training. There are *formative and summative work place based assessments* (WPBA) to assess the development of competencies. Formative WPBA tools (for learning) include formative Objective Structured Assessment of Technical Skills (OSATS) or Specific Learning Events (SLEs), Case-based discussions (CbD) and mini-CEX. The summative assessment (of learning) will be the summative OSATS (Assessment of performance/AoPs). There will be an annual OSATS assessment and the portfolio of evidence has to be submitted for ARCP (Annual Review of Competence Progression). This continues until the achievement of CCT.

One of the critical steps in the training pathway is the progression from basic training to ST-3 (Intermediate training). There are some mandatory requirements for this progression that includes:
- Passing the MRCOG part 1 Exam
- Completing the RCOG Basic Practical Skills course
- Attaining relevant competencies identified in the logbook

The next critical step is the progression to ST-6 (Advanced Training). The mandatory requirements for progression are:
- Passing the MRCOG part 2 and part 3 exam and getting the MRCOG
- Attaining relevant competencies
- Completion of core specialty training modules and ultrasound modules (Fig. 12.2).

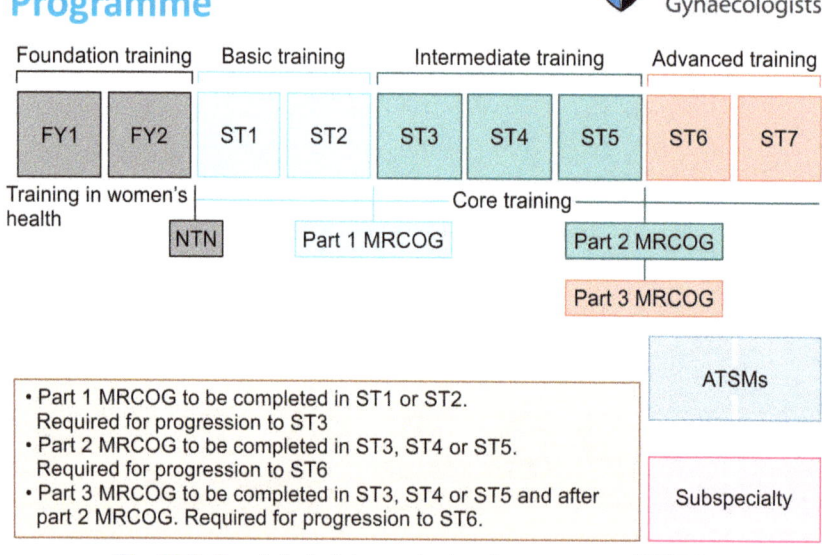

Fig. 12.2: Specialty training and education program of RCOG.

PART 1 MRCOG

Visit the website *rcog.org.uk* and register yourself by creating an account with a username and password. You will be allotted a *college registration* number which you need to quote for all your correspondence with the college.

Go through the exam calendar for part 1. Bookings are open only for a specific time (approximately 4 months prior) for the exam that is conducted twice a year (January and July from 2018).

From 2006, there is no exemptions scheme for part 1 MRCOG. All candidates have to clear all 3 parts to get the membership.

Though only a registered medical degree (MBBS) from a recognized University is required to appear for Part 1 Exam, it is better to have some grounding in postgraduate O&G.

The candidate needs to have eligibility checked before booking a place for the exam.

For this, download the Eligibility Assessment Form from the RCOG website, fill-up and email the completed form with an attached scanned copy of the primary medical degree certificate or degree registration certificate to *part1eligibility@rcog.org.uk*. If you attach a scanned photocopy, it needs to be attested in ink by either a Fellow or a Member or an official of the UK or Indian embassy or a solicitor or public notary.

Currently, the exam fee is £460 for candidates from India.

The exam comprises two written papers each with 100 single best answers (SBAs). Each paper contributes 50% to the total score. There is no minimum score required for each paper and it is only the combined marks of paper 1 and 2 that determines the outcome. The total duration of the exam is 5 hours with a 1 hour lunch break in between.

There are centers in India for both the January (Mumbai, Kolkata) and July (Bangalore, New Delhi) exams.

The syllabus for the Part 1 MRCOG covers the basic and applied sciences relevant to the clinical practice of O&G.

The questions are framed from the modules given in Table 12.1. The standard setting for part 1 MRCOG is done by the Ebel's Method.

Table 12.1: Questions are framed from prescribed modules.

Antenatal care	Management of labor
Clinical skills	Management of delivery
Core surgical skills	Postpartum problems
Early pregnancy care	Postoperative care
Gynecological problems	Surgical procedures
Gynecological oncology	Subfertility
Information technology, clinical governance, research	Sexual and reproductive health
Maternal medicine	Urogynecology and pelvic problems

Ebel's method accounts for the difficulty of each question as well as its relevance to ST3 practice. The method focuses on determining the proportion of borderline candidates who would respond correctly to each exam question. Questions are classified as easy, medium or hard and their relevance is classified as essential, important or acceptable. This creates nine separate categories.

The standard setting panel then decides what percentage of questions they believe a borderline candidate would answer correctly from each category.

If you wish to enter the UK specialists register at any time in the future, you are permitted no more than 6 attempts at the part 1 MRCOG. But for non-UK Trainees with no wish to enter the UK specialists register, there is no limit on attempts.

Learning Resources Recommended by RCOG

e-Learning

- StratOG is RCOG's eLearning platform and contains a SBA resource for Part 1 MRCOG.

To purchase access, email the StratOG team atstratog@rcog.org.uk. It comes to app 44 GBP and is valid for 6 months.

Textbooks

- *Basic Science in O&G* by Philip Bennett and Catherine Williamson
- *Basic Sciences for O&G* by Tim Chard and Richard Lilford
- *Textbook for MRCOG-1* by Basic Sciences in O&G by Richa Saxena
- *Clinical Gynaecological Endocrinology and Infertility* by Fritz, Speroff
- *Last's Anatomy* by Chummy S Sinnatamby
- *Larsen's Humn Embryology* by Schoenwolf, Bleyl, Brauer, Francis
- *Ganong's Medical Physiology* by Barrett, Barman, Baitano, Brooks
- *Harper's Biochemistry* by Murray, Rodwell, Bender, Botham, Weil, Kennelly
- *Robbins Basic Pathology* by Kumar, Abbas, Aster
- *Medical Microbiology* by Murray, Rosenthal, Pfaller
- *Clinical Pharmacology Lecture Notes* by McKay, Walters
- *Essential Medical Genetics* by Tobias, Connor, Smith
- *Statistics at Square 1* by Swinscow, Campbell
- *British National Formulary*
- *MRCOG Part 1: Your Essential Revision Guide* by Fiander, Thilaganathan
- *Revision Notes for the MRCOG Part 1* by Anantharachagan, Sarris, Ugwumadu
- *MRCOG Part 1: Your Essential Revision Guide* by Alison Fiander.

Question Banks

- SBAs for the Part 1 MRCOG by Andrew Sizer, Neil Chapman.

> **Box 12.1:** Tips for MRCOG Part 1 exam.
> - It would be wise not to take the part 1 exam too lightly as there are candidates who have cleared part 2 with relative ease but failed part 1 on their first attempt.
> - Regular focused work for 2 hours a day for 6 months or 4 hours a day for 3 months should see you through.
> - Make a time table and stick to it.
> - One can choose to first brush up on the theory in each module and then attempt the relevant SBAs and EMQs for that module or the other way round. For this just use your MBBS textbooks or borrow new ones from juniors.
> - Subscribe to any one online learning site and attempt all questions in their bank. Make sure you have time for going through the question bank and their explanatory notes at least twice.
> - Note down the points in a notebook for quick revision towards the final phase of preparation.
> - Retain the email you receive when you pass the Part 1 exam as you will not receive any other formal document. You are not allowed to use the letters MRCOG Part 1 against your name.
> - After passing part 1, you should have attempted part 2 at least once in the next 7 years (if you passed after 2013) and at least once within 10 years (if you passed before 2013).

Popular Online Courses

- www.OnExamination.com
- www.BusySpR.com
- Aceonline
- Passmrcog
- CrackingMRCOG.
- www.crackingmrcog.com

Other Popular Question Banks

- SBAs for the MRCOG Part 1 Exam by Gnanasambanthan, Varouxaki, Datta
- Get through MRCOG Part 1 MCQs and EMQs by RekhaWuntakal
- MRCOG Part 1: 400 SBAs by Katherine Andersen
- MRCOG Part 1 Success Manual by Khaldoun Sharif.

(These are available on Amazon.in.) The important tips for Part 1 MRCOG examination are given in Box 12.1.

PART 2 MRCOG

It is a written exam that assesses your knowledge of *obstetrics and gynecology* and the application of your knowledge in clinical scenarios.

From September 2016, the format has been revised. The written exam and oral assessment has been decoupled.

Before applying for the Part 2 MRCOG exam, all candidates are required to have their postregistration (GMC or equivalent Medical Council) training assessed. For this, write to the college quoting your College registration number. You will be sent an Assessment of Training (AoT) form which should be filled up. Certificates on hospital headed paper signed by the Consultants in charge, confirming the nature, grade and dates of the appointments held from graduation/internment has to be attached with the application forms. These certificates are to be attested by a Fellow/Member of RCOG or the University/hospital issuing it or the British Council or Embassy or a Solicitor. Original certificates will not be accepted. There is no fee for this assessment. There are two routes to approval of training:

1. Route A for UK Trainees. UK trainees must be intermediate training (ST-3 or above) to be eligible.
2. Route B for all overseas Candidates. Overseas candidates must demonstrate that they have spent a minimum of 4 years in O&G. This must include at least 2 years (fulltime or equivalent) in O&G within the 4 years preceding a candidate's initial application. All posts overseas, if hospital-based in O&G are now generally accepted. A minimum of 6 months in any single post is required. It usually takes 8 weeks for the AoT application to be processed.

The college will notify the acceptance of eligibility by email and then the candidate can book online for the exam by submitting the entry fees. Applications generally open 5 months before the date of the exam.

There are numerous centers both in UK and around the world where the exam is held twice a year (January and July). Exam fee for candidates in Indian centers is app 427 GBP which can be paid online, by cheque or by bank draft. If you have any doubts, please contact exams@rcog.org.uk.

The entrance tickets are emailed to candidates about 4 weeks before the exam. You need to bring a printout of this along with photographic identification document (e.g. passport). The same rules as for Part 1 exam apply for Part 2. You will lose your exam fee if you withdraw your application after the closing date. If you fail to turn up for the exam, it will not be counted as an attempt.

The Part 2 MRCOG is a written exam with two papers, each for 50% of the total marks. Each paper consists of two question formats—(1) single best answers (SBAs) worth 40% of the total marks and (2) extended matching questions (EMQs) worth 60% of the total marks. The duration is 3 hours for each paper with a 1 hour lunch break. Each paper has 50 SBAs and 50 EMQs.

Standard setting for Part 2 MRCOG is by *Angoff method* wherein a cohort of subject experts evaluate each question and provide an estimate as to how likely the borderline candidate would know the answer. These estimates are averaged and added to a standard error of measurement to determine the final pass mark.

Exam results are emailed directly to the candidates and are no longer put up on the RCOG website. But results may be released to GMC and the respective Deaneries (UK Trainees) and to bonafide third-party enquirers like educational institutions and employers.

As with the Part 1 exam, not more than 6 attempts are allowed at Part 2 for candidates wishing to enter the UK specialist register. For others, there is no limit on the number of attempts. There is also no limit on the length of time between each attempt.

Candidates who pass the Part 2 MRCOG written exam must attempt the Part 3 clinical assessment within 7 years. If not, they will be required to take the Part 2 exam again.

The questions are framed from the modules mentioned for Part 1.

For more detail about content of each module go to Part 2 MRCOG syllabus section or the core curriculum page on the RCOG website (www.rcog.org.uk). You can download the full curriculum for each module there.

Learning Resources Recommended by RCOG for Part 2 MRCOG

Online Resources

- StratOG—RCOG's e-learning platform (core tutorials with SBAs and EMQs)
- RCOG Green Top Guidelines (GTG)
- NICE Guidelines
- RCOG Scientific Impact Papers (SIP)
- The Obstetrician & Gynaecologist (TOG)
- British National Formulary.

Books

- *An Evidence Based Textbook for MRCOG* 3rd edition 2016 by David Leusley, Mark Kilby
- *Bonney's Gynaecological Surgery* 11th edition 2011 by Lopes, Spirtos, Naik, Monaghan
- *Clinical Gynaecological Oncology Ebook 2017* by DiSaia MD, Creasman, Mannel, Scott
- *Contraception Your Questions Answered* 7th edition 2017 by Guillebaud, MacGregor
- *High Risk Pregnancy Management Options* 4th edition 2011 by James, Steer, Weiner, Gonik
- *Handbook of Obstetric Medicine* 5th edition 2015 by Catherine Nelson Piercy
- *Drugs During Pregnancy & Lactation* 3rd edition 2014 by Schaefer, Peters, Miller

- *Martindale: The Complete Drug Reference* 37th edition by RPS, Sean C Sweetman
- *Neonatal-Perinatal Medicine* 9th edition by Martin, Fanaroff, Walsh
- *Dewhurst's Textbook of Obstetrics and Gynaecology* 8th edition 2012 by Keith Edmonds
- *Operative Obstetrics* 2nd edition by Gilstrap, Cunningham, Vandorsten
- *Oxford Speciality Training in O&G* by Sarris, Bewley, Agnihotri.

RCOG and Cambridge University Press Publications

- Fetal Medicine for the MRCOG and Beyond by Cameron, Brennand, Crichton, Gibson
- Gynaecological Oncology for the MRCOG and Beyond by Nigel Acheson, David Leusley
- Management of Infertility for the MRCOG and Beyond by Bhattacharya, Hamilton
- Menopause for the MRCOG and Beyond by Margaret Rees
- Paed Adolescent Gynaecology for MRCOG and Beyond by Garden, Hernon, Topping
- Urogynaecology for MRCOG and Beyond by Price, Jackson
- Reproductive Endocrinology for the MRCOG and Beyond by Adam Balen
- Urodynamics Illustrated by Ranee Thakar, Philip Hobson, Lucia Dolan.

Question Banks

- SBAs for Part 2 MRCOG—Cambridge University Press and RCOG (available on Amazon.in)
- EMQs for MRCOG Part 2 by John Duthie, Paul Hodges.
  Also visit the *Courses and Events Page* on the RCOG website for information on courses run or recommended by the RCOG.

Other Popular and Recommended Learning Resources

Online Resources (Must Read)

- Scottish Intercollegiate Guidelines Network (SIGN) for Gynaec Cancers
- Faculty of Sexual and Reproductive Healthcare Guidelines (FSRH)
- British Association for Sexual Health and HIV Guidelines (BASHH)
- RCOG Consent Advice and Clinical Governance Advice
- RCOG Good Practice, RCOG Statements, Safety alerts
- Joint Guidelines of RCOG with other Royal Colleges
- MBRRACE report (latest)
- NHS Choices
- NHS Cervical Cancer Screening Programme (cancerscreening.nhs.uk/cervical)
- ESHRE Guidelines (Endometriosis, Premature Ovarian Insufficiency).

Popular Question Banks

- SBAs and EMQs for MRCOG II by Chinmayee Ratha, Janesh Gupta
- Practice SBAs for MRCOG Part 2 by Mukhopadhaya Neelanjana
- SBAs and EMQs for MRCOG Part 2 by Shreelata Datta
- SBAs for Part 2 MRCOG by Amanda Jones
- EMQs for the MRCOG Part 2 by Andrea Pilkington
- Get Through MRCOG Part 2: EMQs by Justin Konje
- Part 2 MRCOG: SBA Questions—Andrew Sizer
- MRCOG Part 2: 500 SBAs and EMQs by Rekha Wuntakal
- SBAs for MRCOG Part 2 by Brian Magowan
- Mastering SBA Questions for the Part 2 MRCOG by Adel Elkady.

Online Courses and Groups

- www.drcog-mrcog.info/MRCOG.htm
- www.crackingmrcog.com

Courses in India

- Prof Janesh Gupta's course (Bangalore—January, July)
- Dr Uma Ram's course (Chennai)
- Dr Pranati Reddy's course (Hyderabad).
  The important tips for Part 2 MRCOG examination are given in Box 12.2.

Box 12.2: Tips for MRCOG Part 2 exam.

- There are no shortcuts to clear this exam.
- 5–6 hours of focused study for a minimum of 6 months should see you through. If you are in a busy practice, you may need to spend 2–3 hours a day for a year.
- It would be ideal to have a study partner.
- Choose the study materials wisely and make a timetable.
- It is advisable to attend a couple of courses run in India to get an orientation and a taste of the task ahead.
- Now StratOG is worth spending money on. It has been updated and has almost all materials needed for the exam. It also provides links to refer for further information.
- Be thorough with all the guidelines listed above.
- Subscribe to an online course such as busyspr.Practise EMQs and SBAs relevant to each module from these sites and from question banks daily and write down points from the explanatory notes.
- Join facebook groups such as MRCOG Trademark group which is very useful and clear your doubts by actively taking part in the discussions.
- Make notes from these recommended sources and collect all relevant points for each topic. Arrange notes to fit the modules given in the exam syllabus.
- Keep aside at least 1 month to revise before the exam.
- Book a hotel near the exam venue and reach the previous day.
- Sleep well the night before the exam and do not miss your meals.

PART 3 MRCOG

Once you pass the written Part 2 exam, you can appear for Part 3 Clinical Assessment either immediately or at any time within the next 7 years. Candidates have 4 chances to clear it.

As Part 3 is now a standalone assessment which has been uncoupled from Part 2 written exam, the candidate has to apply online within the published booking window. This opens about 3 months prior to the exam. Keep an eye on the RCOG website (Part 3 exam calendar page) to avoid missing the window. The exam venue can also be chosen at the time of application but the college reserves the right to reallocate the candidate to another exam center due to oversubscription or cancellation of centers.

The fee for candidates from India is 550 GBP. There may be additional administrative fees for some international centers like Singapore.

The hall ticket is usually emailed 4 weeks before the exam.

This exam is a clinical assessment of knowledge, skills, attitude, and competencies. It assesses the following 5 core skill domains.
1. Information gathering
2. Communicating with patients and families
3. Applied clinical knowledge
4. Communicating with colleagues (teamwork)
5. Patient Safety.

The exam consists of 14 tasks which are linked to 14 of the knowledge-based modules given in Table 12.2.

There will be 14 tasks in a circuit. Each task will assess 3–4 domains out of 5 listed earlier. The candidate has 12 minutes to complete each task, which includes 2 minutes of initial reading time.

There will be a trained clinical examiner on all 14 stations and a trained lay examiner on 4 stations. The lay examiner will assess the domains of communication, information gathering, and patient safety.

The candidate can expect two types of tasks mainly:
1. Simulated patient/colleague tasks interacting with a fully briefed trained actor
2. Structured discussion tasks interacting with a clinical examiner.

Table 12.2: Examinations consists of 14 tasks which are linked to 14 of the knowledge-based modules.

Teaching	Postpartum problems
Core surgical skills	Gynecological problems
Postoperative care	Subfertility
Antenatal care	Sexual and reproductive health
Maternal medicine	Early pregnancy care
Management of labor	Gynecological oncology
Management of delivery	Urogynecology and pelvic floor problems

In the first type of task the candidate interacts with an actor who has been trained and fully briefed in the role play, while in the second type of task the examiner will have detailed instructions and a list of questions to guide the discussion.

The candidate is expected to demonstrate the following:
- Convey evidence-based understanding of Part 2 curriculum
- Justify investigations and interventions
- Critically interpret clinical findings and investigation results
  - Critically discuss management options
  - Present a balanced view of risks and benefits of interventions
  - Appropriate introduction and rapport
- Concise and relevant history
- Empathy and active listening
- Manage communication barriers
- Give information in manageable amounts using patient friendly language
- Encourage dialogue and shared decision making
- Demonstrate negotiating skills and respect for patient autonomy
- Acknowledge and address patient's concerns
- Take informed consent, awareness of mental capacity
- Maintain patient dignity
- Ensure use of chaperones
- Sensitive to cultural and religious issues.

As mentioned earlier the number of attempts allowed is 4 (UK and International candidates). If you fail to clear it in 4 attempts, you will need to resit Part 2 exam.

Learning Resources Recommended by RCOG

Online Resources

- StratOG Part 3 elearning (stratog@rcog.org.uk)

Courses

- MRCOG Final Preparation Part 3 Practical course (RCOG)
- Basic Practical Skills in O&G.

Popular Online Courses

- Dr Mustafa's MRCOG Trademark Group-Part 3 course
- Dr Tom McFarlane's tutorials and blog
- Aceonline
- MRCOG Reach
- Success MRCOG

Box 12.3: Tips for MRCOG Part 3 exam.

- In the pre-2016 format you had to sit the OSCE exam 6 weeks after the Part 2 theory exam. This was very difficult for international candidates as there was hardly anytime left to attend courses, practice OSCE stations, and make travel arrangements. So the current format is a welcome change. Though you can choose to sit in the exam immediately after passing Part 2, it would be advisable to sit 6 months later.
- Get a study partner and start practicing stations daily. Revise the Part 2 notes pertaining to each station and scenario. Make a format/template for taking history, doing examination and charting management plans
- Go through all patient information leaflets on RCOG website and learn the way to communicate clearly avoiding medical jargon as majority of stations are counseling stations.
- Keep an eye on the website for the exam booking window.
- Get travel and visa sorted out well in advance.
- Book accommodation preferably near the RCOG office at Regent's park again well in advance as these get booked fast.
- Arrive at least 2 weeks before the exam if you are choosing the London center to get used to the weather as well as to attend a couple of good circuit courses.
- Sleep well on the night before the exam and do not miss your meals.
- Remember Part 3 is not about testing your knowledge alone but it is more to ascertain you are a safe doctor who can work as part of a team, following accepted guidelines and protocols and is a good communicator.
- The key to achieving this gold standard qualification is hard work and practice makes a man perfect.

Textbooks for Part 3

1. *Get through MRCOG:* Arri Coomarasamy and Justin Clark
2. *Part 3 MRCOG: Your Essential Revision Guide:* Lisa Joel, Edmund Neale
3. *OSCEs for the MRCOG Part 2:* Rymer, Hollingworth

Circuit Courses for Part 3 (UK)

1. MRCOG Revision Courses by Teale Fenning
2. Acecourses (Justin Chu, Arri Coomarasamy)
3. Whippscross MRCOG Part 3 Course
4. Part 3 MRCOG Course, St George's Hospital
5. MRCOG Part 3 Course, Whittington Education Centre, London

Circuit Courses in India

1. Bangalore Society—RCOG MRCOG course (Prof Janesh Gupta)
2. TN Society—RCOG MRCOG course (Dr Uma Ram).

The important tips for Part 3 MRCOG examination are given in Box 12.3.

CHAPTER 13

USMLE and Future Prospects

Kajal Parikh

INTRODUCTION

United States of America (USA) is called the land of many dreams and opportunities. It is not surprising that education and residency in the US is the first choice for many doctors from around the world in pursuit of their American dream. This is because statistically:
- USA doctors are paid almost twice as much as Asian and European doctors.
- The opportunities to participate in research, innovations in healthcare and technologic advancement in the field of medicine are one of the best in the world. This leads to an excellent opportunity for professional and personal growth.
- The support of US government for the development of healthcare facilities is the highest worldwide.

This leads to an important question as how to pursue further education for a medical graduate in India and the opportunities thereafter. For any country to practice health care with legal liabilities a government recognized board or professional association is established for standardization of health care practice in the country.

Some such boards for licensing of a medical practitioner in action are:
- United States Medical Licensing Examination (USMLE)—USA
- Medical Council of India (MCI)—India
- Medical Council of Canada Qualifying Examination—Canada
- Professional and Linguistic Assessment Board Test (PLAB)—United Kingdom
- Australian Medical Council (AMC)—Australia
- Ärztliche Prüfungen (IMPP)—Germany
- Dubai Health Authority (DHA)—Dubai
- Saudi Medical Licensing Examination (SMLE)—Saudi Arabia
- Nepal Medical Council—Nepal, and many more.

UNITED STATES MEDICAL LICENSING EXAMINATION

It is a licensing board in the United States for Health Care Professionals. Any medical graduate outside of the United States is referred to as International

Medical Graduate (IMG) and has to take USMLE for practice of medicine in the US.

USMLE is supervised and cosponsored by:
- National Board of Medical Education (NBME) for US or Canadian Medical Graduates.
- Federation of State Medical Boards (FSMB)
- Education Commission for Foreign Medical Graduates (ECFMG).

ECFMG specifically looks after all the non-US medical graduates (IMG/FMGs). For IMGs, the candidate first has to apply for a membership on the NBME website that will direct you to ECFMG website. The candidate will then get to apply and pay for USMLE examination.

The eligibility for ECFMG certification is follows:
- Step 1
- Step 2 CK
- Step 2 CS

Pass—maximum 6 *attempts each* but within *7-year* period of passing any first USMLE Step

Prior to Applying

The candidate must formulate strategy and goals based on simple facts and statistics:
- USMLE tests are friendlier with fresh graduates than senior pass outs.
- Higher the scores, better are the chances (>230).
- Improve one's language skills and acculturation.
- The student has to be a part of a medical school that has met with ECFMG eligibility criteria listed on ECFMG website.
- The specialties comfortable with recruiting IMG are:
  - Internal Medicine
  - Pediatrics
  - Psychiatry
  - Family Medicine
- However, a combination of high score, good clinical skillsets, strong resume and consistent research work can lead to residency in:
  - Anesthesiology
  - Obstetrics and Gynecology
  - General Surgery
  - Orthopedic Surgery
- NBME practice tests and USMLE: *World and Kaplan Pretest* are recommended to prepare for USMLE examinations.
- Resume building by various academic opportunities in the desired specialty can be targeted. A publication in peer-reviewed scientific journal, clinical trial participation in home country can significantly increase the chances of a match.

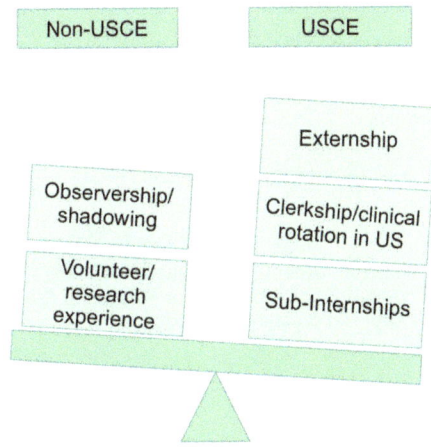

Fig. 13.1: US clinical experience.

What is US Clinical Experience?

- *USMLE during Internship:* Opt for externship/clerkship during the course of internship (Fig. 13.1).
- *USMLE for post-MBBS graduate:* Opt for a sub-internship in the field or hospital of their choice.
- *USMLE for post-MD/MS-ObGyn:* Opt for a researcher's post/observers post in various departments of OBGYN.
- Working as a volunteer/or in support group in collaboration with US hospitals.
- *How to apply*
  - Contacting hospitals for direct placements.
  - Using paid placements.
  - Residency forums/hospital websites/facebook page.
- Benefits
  - US-based letters of recommendation.
  - Connections in US medical world.
  - Strong electronic residency application service (ERAS) application for residency.

Options for International Medical Graduates (Fig. 13.2)

- MD in USA after MBBS in India
- MD in USA after MBBS in Caribbean
- MD in USA after MBBS in India + MPH in USA.

Course Details

United States Medical Licensing Examination is a three-step process irrespective of the medical credentials in one's home country (Fig. 13.3).

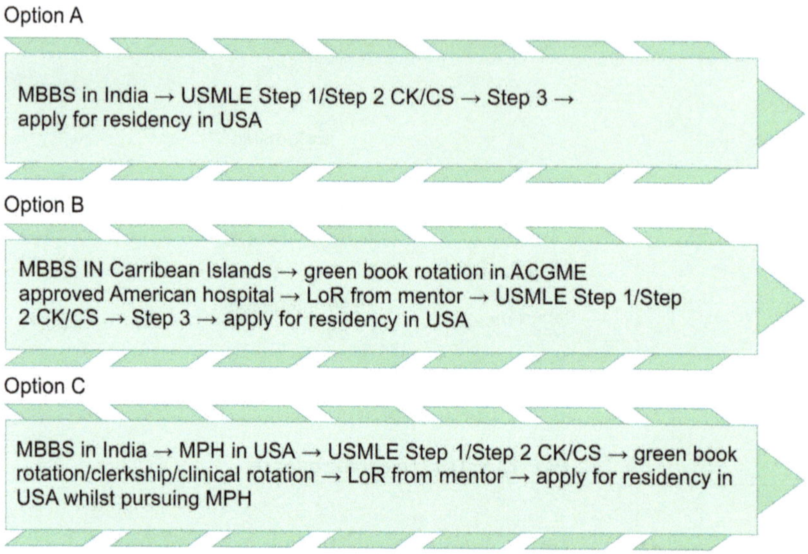

Option A
MBBS in India → USMLE Step 1/Step 2 CK/CS → Step 3 → apply for residency in USA
Option B
MBBS IN Carribean Islands → green book rotation in ACGME approved American hospital → LoR from mentor → USMLE Step 1/Step 2 CK/CS → Step 3 → apply for residency in USA
Option C
MBBS in India → MPH in USA → USMLE Step 1/Step 2 CK/CS → green book rotation/clerkship/clinical rotation → LoR from mentor → apply for residency in USA whilst pursuing MPH

Fig. 13.2: Options for international medical graduate (IMG).

USMLE Step 1, Step 2 (CK/CS), Step 3
ECFMG certification
Interviews and residency match

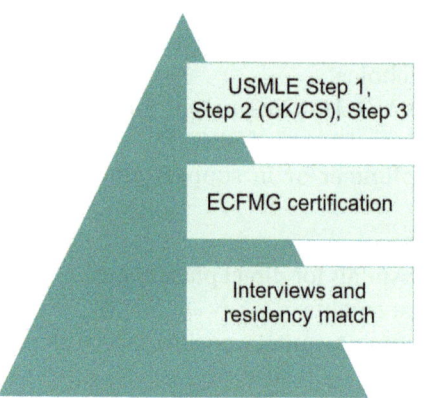

Fig. 13.3: Three-step process of United States Medical Licensing Examination (USMLE) course.

USMLE is a *multiple choice question* licensing examination universally taken by all medical graduates passed out from and outside the United States.

The three step process is complementary to one another and cannot be skipped or avoided for attaining the medical license to practice.

USMLE Steps

USMLE Step 1

Step 1 in USMLE assesses the knowledge of a medical student in Basic Sciences and its medical and clinical application.

Subjects in Step 1 are:
1. Anatomy
2. Biochemistry
3. Physiology
4. Pathology
5. Pharmacology
6. Microbiology
7. Behavioral Sciences
8. *Others:* Nutrition, Aging Genetics.

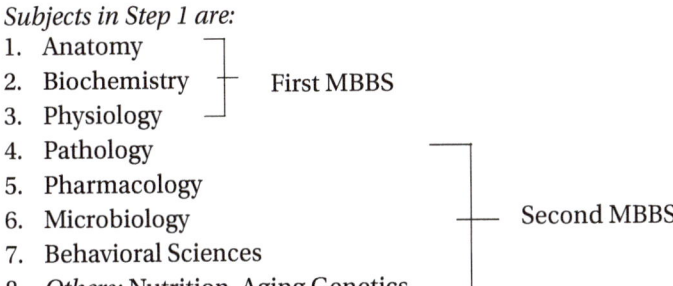

Step 1 format: Seven slots of strict one hour each over an eight hour period with approximately 35–40 questions (total of 280 questions).

USMLE Step 2

It consists of two parts:
1. *USMLE Step 2 Clinical Knowledge (CK):* Step 2 CK is an assessment of clinical knowledge and skills and its medical application.
   Subjects in STEP 2 CK are:
   1. Ophthalmology
   2. Preventive Medicine
   3. Medical Ethics
   4. Internal Medicine
   5. Surgery
   6. Pediatrics
   7. Obstetrics and Gynecology
   8. Dermatology
   9. Radiology
   10. Psychiatry
   11. Emergency Medicine

   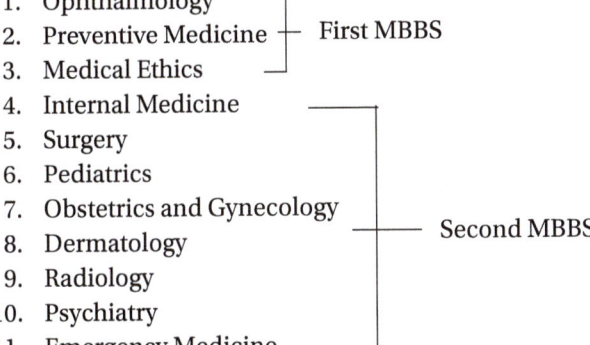

   USMLE Step 2 format: Eight slots of strict one hour each over a nine hour period with approximately 35–40 questions (total of 318 questions).
2. *USMLE Step 2 Clinical Skills (CS):* Step 2 CS in USMLE is for medical graduates to test their clinical and communication skills and command over English language and patient-centric application of medical knowledge. The student has to follow basic medical protocols and principles of counseling during the course of this test.
   Format of Exam:
   - 12 dummy patients over 8 hours.
   - 15 min of patient encounter for history and examination.
   - 10 min to record the history on computer.

   The examination is only offered in the following cities across USA and nowhere else in the world:
   - Philadelphia
   - Chicago

- Atlanta
- Houston
- Los Angeles.

Facts of Step 1 and Step 2:
- Step 1 and Step 2 CK/CS is mandatory for applying for residency in the US can be taken in any sequence.
- Step 3 can be taken only when a student has passed Step 1/Step 2CK-CS.
- Once a student *passes* the examination, the results are permanently recorded and there is no option to retake the test for a choice of a different score.
- Failed attempts are documented and maximum of six failed attempts are allowed. A test cannot be repeated for more than three times in a 12-month period.
- If a student does not pass or appear for all the required steps within a 7-year-period that begins from the date of first ever USMLE Step appeared, then after the 7 years—all the previously appeared USMLE tests and scores are deemed invalid and the candidate has to start with a new account and reappear for all the tests again.
- Step 1/Step 2 CK is a single day examination with fixed time frames at prefixed Prometric centers in the city of choice listed on the official website all around the world.
- A total cumulative of one hour of break time can be divided in any way the candidate desires ranging between 5 min and 15 min.

USMLE Step 3—FSMB Registration

Step 3 is a 2-day examination:
- *Day 1:* Foundation in Independent Practice (FIP). Concepts tested— scientific principles for basic medical care.
  - Duration: One day—7 hours, 6 slots of one hour each with 35–40 questions. Total of 260 questions.
- *Day 2:* Advanced Clinical Medicine (ACM). Concept tested—applying medical knowledge to patient management.
  - Duration: One day—9hrs, 6 slots of 45 minute with 30 questions.

A total of 180 questions. Also, there are 13 case simulations, 10–20 minute each.

The details of USMLE examination are given in Table 13.1.

APPLICATION PROCESS

After the tests the candidate has to make an *ERAS* account for registering for National Resident Matching Program (NRMP). *NRMP* provides 3Rs— *registration/ranking/results* and is what connects the residency program to

Table 13.1: USMLE exam details.

	Fees in dollars	Location	When can they be taken?	Average preparation time	Pass/average score
Step 1	$630 + Regional surcharge	India/USA at any Prometric Test Center	Can be given during MBBS (Usually in Third MBBS or after Internship)	6–8 months	194/229
Step 2 CK	$630 + Regional surcharge	INDIA/USA at any Prometric Test Center	Can be given during MBBS (Usually after Internship)	6 months	209/240
Step 2 CS	$1,290	USA on Visitors Visa (5 listed cities)	Preferred after Step 1 and Step 2 CK	1 month	Pass/Fail
Step 3	$850	USA on Visitors Visa	Always after Step 1/Step 2CK/CS	4 months	196

applicants. It is applicable for all immigrant and non-immigrant students applying for residency for a particular year. All their credentials are registered with NRMP and are highly secured and confidential. The process for application starts from mid-September and continues until December 31st. Applications sent earlier are better and response is proven better before October 31st. The NRMP exchanges data with ECFMG to recertify the status of IMG. Hence, only the students who are eligible to begin training on July 1 in the year of the match will be allowed to participate.

Documents for Application

- ERAS account for every student
- Complete resume
- ECFMG report and USMLE transcripts
- Proof of graduation from home country including medical transcripts/letter from Dean.
- A cover letter for each program and specialty addressed to the director of respective program explaining why you are the right fit for that particular program and specialty.
- A *personal statement* describing why should a program select you against all the other applicants.
- Letters of recommendation—from home country/US accredited hospitals, doctors, and research assistants.

- *Exception to the rule:* State of California along with the above it requires "Applicant Evaluation Status Letter"—issued and certified by California Medical Board. This is not IMG friendly.
- The trick is to attend residency fairs listed on American Academy of Family Physicians (AAFP).

IMG Friendly Programs

Apply in as many IMG friendly programs as possible (25-80) that are listed on the website. The more the programs you apply, the more are the chances of getting called for an interview. IMG friendly states and IMG friendly specialities keep varying and are updated after each NRMP on the website.

Interview

- Once you receive an email stating the acceptance for an interview, read about the hospital; its working style and the motto of the institute.
- Respond back promptly, completely and professionally.
- Dress appropriately and conduct yourself with grace.
- Behave professionally with every person you encounter at the institute. Everyone including receptionist could evaluate your behavior.
- After the interview, a directed "Thank you" email to the Program Director within the first 48 hr can show your inclination and interest toward the program and reinstate your personality in the program directors mind.
- After interviewing at different universities all over United States the candidate submits a list of preference of his/her institutes on NRMP website.
- A similar list is submitted by the Program Director of the Institutes who have interviewed and the NRMP runs an *automated match*.
- A particular date is set for "the match" when a student gets to know where they are going to go for further studies.

Don'ts

- As lucrative as health care can get there are companies that exploit IMGs. Recognize and avoid them. They provide paid clerkships with mediocre doctors and send electronic copies of your application to any and every program without a good reputation for guaranteeing admission.

To Obtain a Visa

International Medical Graduates who are not citizens or lawful permanent residents must obtain valid visa for pursuing residency in the US.

Most commonly acquired non-immigrant visas for doctors planning to practice and live in the United States are:

J-1 Visa: ECFMG sponsored Exchange Visitor Visa for duration of Residency. J-1 visa holders need to return to their home country for a minimum of 2 years before returning to the US. However most students can get their J-1 waiver available by
- Obtaining a *no-objection letter/statement* from the government of country of origin
- Conrad Waiver
- Persecution Waiver or Hardship Waiver wherein wife or child is a green-card holder or citizen.
- *Interested Government Agency Waiver (IGA):* By working in Health Professional Shortage Area (HPSA)

H1-B Visa: Temporary Worker Visa sponsored by the institute hiring you at every step of the way.

H-3 Visa: Only for training purpose. The doctor cannot overstay the period of visa or training.

O-1 Visa: Whereby doctors possess extraordinary skillset proven by physician of the respective field.

Down the road of residency and after, one can become eligible to pursue legitimate, permanent residency in the United States.

RETURN TO INDIA AFTER MD IN USA

American residency and fellowship is accepted by the MCI in India and one can practice as a specialist in India without clearing any additional examinations.

The biggest hurdle is the difference in the approach to management of a patient, the doctor-patient relationship and the quality of life provided in India as opposed to the United States.
- Payment during residency: Stipend during Residency is $45,000–$60,000 per annum
- Hours of work: An average resident works around 60–80 hours/week including ancillary work.

Obstetrics and Gynecology

The average obstetrics and gynecology salary across United States for consultants is given in Figure 13.4.

Exception

The Federation of State Medical Boards can also provide temporary licensing in OBGYN for that particular university for a brief period of time without USMLE licensing of the candidate.

108 Exploring New Horizons in Obstetrics and Gynecology

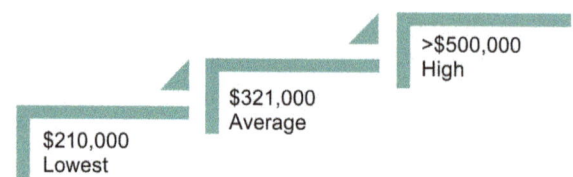

Fig. 13.4: Average obstetrics and gynecology salary across United States for consultants.

Malpractice Insurance

Malpractice insurance is extremely important and paramount importance for legal coverage during medical practice. It is the highest for obstetricians and gynecologist ranging from $85,000 per annum to $200,000 per annum.

FELLOWSHIPS

Fellowship after postgraduation in India requires an application process that begins 18 months before the fellowship commences along with USMLE examinations (Table 13.2).

Fellowships are available in:
- Family Planning
- Gynecologic Oncology
- Maternal-Fetal Medicine
- Reproductive Endocrinology and Infertility
- Minimal Access Surgery and Robotic Surgery
- Female Pelvic Medicine and Reconstructive Surgery.

Table 13.2: Application process for getting fellowship after postgraduation.		
Months	Activity	Documents
December (previous year)	Registration for fellowship commences	Application forms
February (current year)	Registration for fellowship ends	Letters of recommendation
March (current year)	Interview commences	Travel to universities for interviews
May (current year)	Submit each candidates rank order listing (ROL)	Weigh the preference of the fellowship and university where you interviewed
June (current year)	Announcement of fellowship match/scramble	Confirm/Reject
August (next year)	Fellowship begins	

The duration of fellowship is between 2 years and 3 years and after completion of fellowship one can apply for an attending consultant position at institute of choice.

The residency program in the United States is centralized with all the residents in the country getting the same standardized training. The better and organized living conditions in the United States, advanced technological paradigm, newer research based advances, funds, and resources for investigation and advancement and better quality of life allures the best of medical school student to pursue the road of USMLE for defining their future. The need to assess long-term goals, personality, social and financial responsibility and personality and attitude of the candidate is of paramount importance. It rightly puts to practice, when the going gets tough, the tough get going!

BIBLIOGRAPHY

1. American Academy of Family Physicians. [online] Available from https://www.aafp.org/home.html. [Accessed November, 2018].
2. American Academy of Family Physicians. Medical School Residency. [online] Available from https://www.aafp.org/medical-school-residency/residency/apply/img.html. [Accessed November, 2018].
3. American Medical Association. [online] Available from https://www.ama-assn.org. [Accessed November, 2018].
4. American Medical Colleges. [online] Available from https://www.amc.org/services/eras/. [Accessed November, 2018].
5. Association of American Medical Colleges. [online] Available from https://students-residents.aamc.org. [Accessed November, 2018].
6. Educational Commission for Foreign Medical Graduates. [online] Available from https://www.ecfmg.org. [Accessed November, 2018].
7. Educational Commission for Foreign Medical Graduates. Frequent Questions. [online] Available from https://iwa2.ecfmg.org/iwafaq.asp. [Accessed November, 2018].
8. Federation of State Medical Boards of the United States. [online] Available from http://www.fsmb.org/step-3. [Accessed November, 2018].
9. Fellowship Era. [online] Available from https://www.erasfellowshipdocuments.org. [Accessed November, 2018].
10. National Board of Medical Examiners®. [online] Available from https://www.nbme.org. [Accessed November, 2018].
11. National Resident Matching Program. [online] Available from http://www.nrmp.org. [Accessed November, 2018].
12. Prometric. [online] Available from https://www.prometric.com. [Accessed November, 2018].
13. United States Medical Licensing Examination®. [online] Available from https://www.usmle.org. [Accessed November, 2018].

Cosmetic Gynecology: An Overview

Deepa Ganesh

INTRODUCTION

Great advances have been made over the past several decades to enhance men's sexual needs, both medical and surgical. Injections, implants and the recent use of *Viagra* have addressed male issues of impotence and erectile dysfunction. Women on a general note do not pay too much attention to the physical aspects of sexuality. In a woman's life physiologic changes such as childbirth, hormonal changes due to aging and menopause, weight fluctuations may alter the laxity of the vaginal canal, devitalize the mucosal tone of the vaginal wall and damage the pelvic floor, These often lead to the development of genitourinary conditions such as vaginal atrophy, dryness, stress urinary incontinence, and physiologic distress affecting a woman's self-confidence, sexuality and quality of life. Various treatment modalities were available to manage these indications, varying from invasive vaginal surgery to more benign treatments like topical vaginal hormonal gels or hormone-replacement therapy.

Cosmetic gynecology is the new kid on the block in the esthetic field that changes female external genitalia appearance to look more natural and younger (Fig. 14.1). The procedures in this specialty are done either to improve the appearance or boost up function or both. This is one of the fastest growing surgical procedures, with women increasingly realizing that they do not have to simply accept something that is making them unhappy.

HISTORY

First evidence on female genital modification dates back to around 163 BC from the ancient Egyptian civilization.[1] Since then it is known that women have modified their genitals with adornments, bleaches, reductive and expansive techniques.

Gynecological surgeons have performed surgical procedures for altering the size, appearance and function of the female genitals for several years. But these procedures have aimed to repair genitals after obstetrical delivery, in intersex or transgender persons and in case of pediatric labial hypertrophy.

Chapter 14: Cosmetic Gynecology: An Overview 111

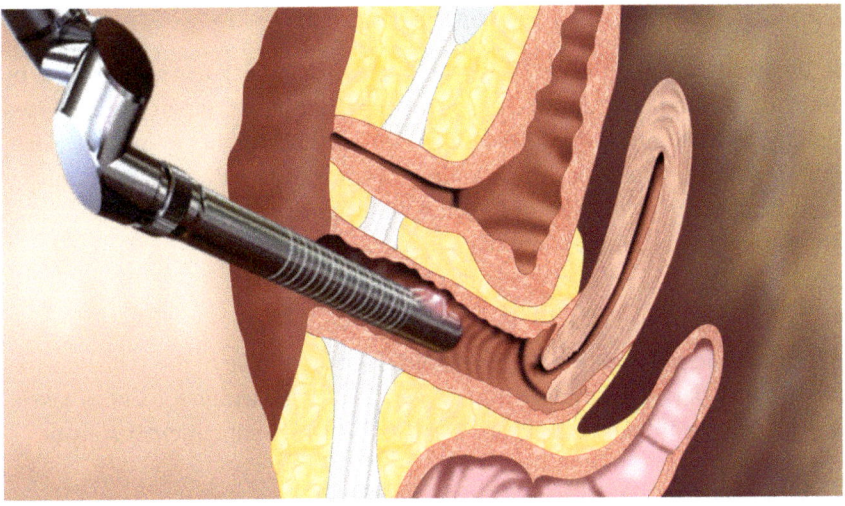

Fig. 14.1: Nonsurgical vaginal tightening.

Honore and O'Hara in 1978,[2] Hodgekinson and Hait,[3] Chavis, LaFeria and Niccolin in 1989[4] were the first to describe female genital surgeries performed for esthetic purposes and for sexual enhancement.

Although late 1980s witnessed the publishing of multiple articles on vulvar labiaplasty technique and small retrospective case series, it was not until the 21st century that procedures designed specifically for reduction of labial and clitoral hood size, narrowing of the hymenal aperture, and increasing vaginal wall pressure by surgical narrowing of the vagina were widely discussed over internet and published in press.

A major milestone was an article by Gary Alter in 1998. Through the article Alter reported the "modified V-wedge" technique for reducing labial volume. It supposedly had better cosmetic outcome and lesser risk of neurological injury when compared to the linear resection based labiaplasty which was performed prior to that time.

David Matlock is one of the early pioneers in the field of female genital plastic surgery. To his credit is the development of Laser assisted techniques namely *designer laser vaginoplasty and laser vaginal rejuvenation.* During early days of his research into the subject, he carefully laid down guidelines in relation to clinical practice and patient selection.

SURGICAL PROCEDURES IN COSMETIC GYNECOLOGY

Female genital plastic surgery is surgery on the female external genitalia and vagina designed to subjectively improve appearance, diminish discomfort, and/or potentially provides psychological and functional improvement in sexual stimulation and satisfaction.

Labiaplasty or Labia Minora Reduction

It involves conservative excision of the excess labial tissue followed by suturing of the labial edges. The various techniques of repair are Sculpted linear resection, wedge resection, de-epithelization, W-plasty, laser labiaplasty, custom flask, fenestration and composite reduction technique.[5,6] The surgical repair may be performed with the help of instruments such as stem-iris scissors, scalpel or contact laser.

Labia Majora Reduction

Majora reduction involves vertical excision of an ellipse of the labial dermis along with a part of the underlying adipose tissue lying within the Colles' fascia. It is followed by repair using monofilament 3-0 to 5-0 subcuticular sutures.

Labia Majora Augmentation

This procedure provides esthetically enhanced and youthful labia majora by autologous fat transfer or by fillers and platelet rich plasma (PRP).

Clitoral Hood Reduction

It is generally performed for reduction of redundant preputial tissue. The redundant tissue is excised unilaterally or bilaterally depending on the need. The excision should be performed well lateral to the underlying clitoral shaft. Care should be taken to remain superficial so as to avoid damaging the dorsal nerve of clitoris which enters anterolaterally.

Mons Reduction

It involves reduction of the fat tissue of the mons pubis. The excessive adipose tissue deep to the superficial fascia is accessed and removed. Large blood vessels may be encountered during the process and hemostasis should be achieved adequately with electrocautery or ligation.

Hymenoplasty

It is commonly known as a "revirgination" procedure. Hymenoplasty involves making two or more diamond shaped excisions, with the widest part of the diamond just inside the hymenal ring and the external apex pointing to the vestibule. Later each excision is closed vertically using fine absorbable sutures to result in a smaller and tight hymenal aperture.

Vaginal Rejuvenation

Vaginal rejuvenation is a blanket term used to describe procedures done to tighten the vaginal canal and to elevate and strengthen the perineal body so as to improve female vaginal sexual sensation. Vaginal rejuvenation includes perineoplasty and vaginoplasty. They are modifications of traditional colporrhaphy.[7] Laser vaginal rejuvenation uses laser for cutting and dissecting, and employs sutures to tighten the muscles of the vagina. It can also treat stress incontinence apart from enhancing sexual gratification.

Designer Laser Vaginoplasty

It is a comprehensive set of procedures designed by David Matlock with the aim to beautify the female external genitalia and heighten sexual pleasure. It includes:
- Laser reduction of excess prepuce
- Laser reduction of labia minora with reduction of labia minora thickness
- Liposculpturing of the mons pubis and labia majora
- Laser reduction of labia majora
- Labia majora augmentation via fat transfer or fillers
- Suprapubic lift of vulvar structures.

NONSURGICAL PROCEDURES

G-Spot Augmentation

It is a technique first described by David Matlock in 2002. It is an outpatient procedure which involves injecting human high molecular weight hyaluronic acid in the Grafenberg spot (G-spot) which is a highly erogenous area in the anterior vaginal wall.[8] It temporarily augments G-Spot in sexually active women with normal sexual function. The procedure is performed under local anesthesia. The injection may need to be repeated every 4–6 months for sustained results.

Orgasm Shot

This outpatient procedure, invented by Charles Runels in 2011, treats sexual dysfunction and improves orgasm by injecting autologous platelet rich plasma (PRP) around the clitoris, orgasm shot (O-Spot) and vagina. These platelets then activate the growth of new cells in the injected areas, making that part more sensitive to the touch and hence vaginal and clitoral rejuvenation.[9]

Laser Vaginal Tightening

This procedure involves application of nonsurgical CO_2 or Erbium Laser probe in the vaginal canal which apply thermal energy to the various layers of the vaginal tissue, stimulating collagen regeneration contracture of elastin fibers and neovascularization which results in thickening and tightening of the vaginal walls and urethra to improve atrophy and urine loss.[10]

Laser Vulval and Vaginal Skin Lightening

It removes darker pigmentation around the vaginal and perineum area. The skin is treated with low potency topical steroids 2–3 days prior to laser treatment.[11]

ETHICAL CONSIDERATIONS

The demand for female genital cosmetic procedures has been on the high over the past few years. In such a scenario it is important for the surgeons to abide by certain ethics while providing cosmetic gynecology services.

The first of the few central ethical principles is autonomy. Autonomy confers upon a person the right to decide whether or not to have a procedure done. For complete autonomy it is important for the person to be free from coercive influences and to have a detailed understanding of the risks, benefits and alternatives of any treatment. This can be ensured by obtaining an informed consent.[12]

Nonmaleficence meaning "do no harm" is another important ethical consideration. It is important when a surgical procedure is done purely for esthetic purposes. Though surgical complications are not always completely avoidable, established procedures performed by surgeons with expertise may have lower complication rates.

The ultimate benefits of a procedure to the patient can be determined only by finding out the motivation of a patient to undergo the procedure.

If the investment put into developing cosmetic genital surgery is not justifiable considering limited medical resources of a community, it may end up in the list of unethical medical practices.

Whom to Operate

- Educated, informed patients, who understand their alternatives or uneducated who are educated with their problems.
- Patients who are considering surgery *for themselves,* not only to "please" their sexual partner, although that desire may reasonably be part of the equation.[13]
- Patients with reasonable expectations.
- Patients for whom this is not a "spur of the moment" decision!
- It can be safely performed any time after sexual maturity (minimum patient age of 18 year).

Whom not to Operate

- Active gynecological disease, such as infection or malignancy.
- Smokers, poorly controlled diabetics, uncontrolled hypertensives, tuberculosis and other medical illness.

- Patients with "body dysmorphic disorder", psychosis or anxiety disorder.
- Patients who may have unreasonable expectations.
- Patient who get a picture and say "look exactly like *"that"*.

OPPORTUNITIES IN COSMETIC GYNECOLOGY

As alluded to already, *cosmetic gynecology* is an evolving subspecialty. Though there are no epidemiological studies looking at the prevalence of these issues in India, going by statistics from the west, the need for this specialty is expected to increase in the future. Considering the day care approach, the nonsurgical modalities of treatment, quick recuperation and reduced morbidity, cosmetic gynecology could become an integral part of the armamentarium for most if not all gynecologists. Cost of laser machines may dampen interest for some time though. However, with more companies pitching in and with more participation from gynecologists, the future might augur well for this nascent subspecialty.

International Society of Cosmetogynecology and European Society of Aesthetic Gynecology to name a few, are the organizations offering guidance on training and certification in the field of *cosmetic gynecology.*

CONCLUSION

Beauty is every woman's desire, be it even the most intimate areas. Sometimes a woman may feel unhappy with the appearance of her genitals and face body image issues. It may have psychosexual impact on the woman.

Also as a woman goes through childbirth, aging, weight fluctuations and hormonal changes nearing menopause, the elasticity and youthfulness of her genitalia get affected. The genital tissues become loose and may sag causing them to be unsightly. Vaginal laxity may also reduce sexual pleasure.

Recent developments in the field of female genital cosmetic surgery has come as a boon to many women who wish to give themselves a chance at transforming their bodies to look sexually more appealing and to be able to experience heightened sexual gratification.

The outcome of the procedures may be highly variable though, depending on many factors such as the woman's expectation, general medical condition of the patient, the expertise of the surgeon, psychosexual status of the patient, etc.

REFERENCES

1. Goodman MP, Placik O, Matlock D. Female genital plastic and cosmetic surgery. Philadelphia: Wiley-Blackwell; 2016. pp. 3-8.
2. Honore LH, O'Hara KE. Benign enlargement of the labia minora. Eur J Obstet Gynaecol Reprod Biol. 1978;8:61-4.

3. Hodgekinson DJ, Hait G. Aesthetic vaginal labiaplasty. Plast Reconst Surg. 1984;74:414-6.
4. Chavis WM, LaFeria JJ, Niccolin IR. Plastic repair of elongated hypertrophic labia minora: a case report. J Reprod Med. 1989;34:3737-45.
5. Alter GJ. A new technique for aesthetic labia minora reduction. Ann Plast Surg. 1998;40:287-90.
6. Oranges CM, Sisti A, Sisti G. Labia minora reduction techniques: a comprehensive literature review. Aesth Surg J. 2015;35(4):419-31.
7. Pardo JS, Sola VD, Ricci PA, et al. Colpoperineoplasty in women with a sensation of a wide vagina. Acta Obstet Gynaecol Scand. 2006;85:1125-7.
8. Addiego F, Belzer EG, Comolli J, et al. Female ejaculation: a case study. J Sex Res. 1981;17:13-21.
9. Runels C, Melnick H, Debourbon E, et al. A pilot study of the effect of localized injections of autologous platelet rich plasma (PRP) for the treatment of female sexual dysfunction. J Women Heal Care. 2014;3:169.
10. Karcher C, Sadick N. Vaginal rejuvenation using energy based devices. Int J Women Dermatol. 2016;2(3):85-8.
11. Hunzeker C. Fractionated CO_2 laser resurfacing: our experience with more than 2,000 treatments. Aesth Surg J. 2009:29;401-16.
12. Garrett TM, Baillie HW. Health care ethics: principles and problems, 2nd edition. Upper Saddle River, New Jersey: Prentice Hall; 1993.
13. Goodman MP, Placik OJ, Benson RH et al. A large multicentre outcome study of female genital plastic surgery. J Sex Med. 2010;7:1565-77.

CHAPTER 15

Civil Services (IAS/IPS)

Sarveshwar Bhure, Shailesh Balkawade

INTRODUCTION

The Civil Services Examination is a competitive examination in India conducted by the Union Public Service Commission (UPSC) for recruitment to various Civil Services of the Government of India, including the Indian Administrative Service (IAS), Indian Foreign Service (IFS), Indian Police Service (IPS), etc. Also simply referred as UPSC examination.

The District Collector is a bureaucrat of the IAS. The district Superintendent of Police (SP) is an IPS Officer. The tax collection is the duty of Indian Revenue Service (IRS) officer. They are responsible for public affairs in the entire district of a State. They are recruited by the Central Government of India. It is their task to handle the law and order of that particular district, collect the revenue and taxation. These civil service officers form the backbone of the Indian system of Governance. They are the implementing authority and the directly answerable to the system.

SERVICES

Civil services examination is conducted by the UPSC. Following are the services which one gets on qualifying the examination.

All India Services

- Indian Administrative Service
- Indian Police Service
- Indian Forest Service.

Central Services (Group A)

- Indian Post and Telecommunication Accounts and Finance Service (IP & TAFS)
- Indian Audit and Accounts Service (IA & AS)
- Indian Civil Accounts Service (ICAS)
- Indian Corporate Law Service (ICLS)
- Indian Defence Accounts Service (IDAS)

- Indian Defence Estates Service (IDES)
- Indian Foreign Service
- Indian Information Service (IIS)
- Indian Ordnance Factories Service (IOFS)
- Indian Postal Service (IPoS)
- Indian Railway Accounts Service (IRAS)
- Indian Railway Personnel Service (IRPS)
- Indian Railway Traffic Service (IRTS)
- Indian Revenue Service (IRS-IT)
- Indian Revenue Service (IRS-C & CE)
- Indian Trade Service (ITrS)
- Railway Protection Force (RPF).

Group B Services

- Armed Forces Headquarters Civil Services (AFHCS)
- Delhi, Andaman and Nicobar Islands Civil Service (DANICS)
- Delhi, Andaman and Nicobar Islands Police Service (DANIPS)
- Pondicherry Civil Service (PCS)
- Pondicherry Police Service (PPS).

ROLES AND RESPONSIBILITIES

The *role of IAS officers* is very dynamic, demands a great deal of responsibility and reverence. The responsibilities of an IAS officer are:
- Handling affairs of government that involve framing and implementation of policy.
- Implementing policies through supervision and at grass root levels.
- Disbursement of funds through personal supervision.
- IAS officers join the state administration at the subdivisional level, resuming their services as subdivisional magistrates, and look after law and order, general administration and development work in the area assigned to them.
- The post of the District Officer also known as District Magistrate, District Collector or Deputy Commissioner is the highly respected and responsible post the IAS officers enjoy.
- At the district level, an IAS officer deals with district affairs, including implementation of developmental programs.
- The officers may also be appointed in the State Secretariat or they may serve as Heads of Departments or in Public Sector Undertakings.
- At the Center, IAS officers serve at the highest position as the Cabinet Secretaries, Secretaries/Additional Secretaries, Joint Secretaries, Directors, Deputy Secretaries and Under Secretaries.

- At the Center, the IAS officers play a key role in formulation and implementation of policies related to a particular area; for instance, finance, commerce, etc.

Indian Police Service Officer is the heart of Law and Order situation of the country. Their functions are:
- To fulfill duties in the areas of maintenance of public peace and order, crime prevention, investigation, and detection, collection of intelligence, very important person (VIP) security, border policing, railway policing, smuggling, drug trafficking, economic offences, corruption in public life, disaster management, enforcement of socioeconomic legislation, biodiversity and protection of environmental laws, etc.
- IPS officer joins the service as Sub-Divisional Police Officer (SDPO) in a district and is incharge of one or more talukas. Before that, he also works at the grass root level as the Officer Incharge (OI).
- Superintendent of Police heads the police force of a district. They are entrusted with the powers and responsibility of maintaining law and order and related issues of a district of a state or a union territory (UT) of India. Their rank badge is the Ashoka emblem above one star. The equivalent post in metro (Commissionerate) is Deputy Commissioner of Police (DCP).
- IPS officers play a role in leading and commanding the Indian Intelligence Agencies like Research and Analysis Wing (RAW), Intelligence Bureau (IB), Central Bureau of Investigation (CBI), Criminal Investigation Department (CID), etc.
- Indian Federal Law Enforcement Agencies, Civil and Armed Police Forces in all the states and UTs.
- IPS officers also play a role in leading and commanding the Central Armed Police Forces (CAPF) which include the Central Police Organisations (CPO) such as Border Security Force (BSF), Central Reserve Police Force (CRPF), Indo-Tibetan Border Police (ITBP), National Security Guard (NSG), Central Industrial Security Force (CISF), Vigilance Organisations and Indian Federal Law Enforcement Agencies.
- Serve at managerial/policy making levels in the Ministries and Departments of Central and State governments and public sector undertakings both at center and states, and the RAW, Government of India.
- With courage, uprightness, dedication and a strong sense of service to the people, IPS Officers lead/command the force.
- Inculcate integrity of the highest order, sensitivity to aspirations of people in a fast-changing social and economic milieu, respect for human rights, broad liberal perspective of law and justice, high standard of professionalism, physical fitness and mental alertness.

HOW TO PREPARE FOR THE EXAMINATION?

It has three parts:
1. *Preliminary examination*: Preliminary examination, now popularly known as the Civil Services Aptitude Test (CSAT) (officially it is still called General Studies Paper-1 and Paper-2), intends to focus on analytical abilities and understanding rather than the ability to memorize. The new pattern includes two papers of two hours duration and 200 marks each.
2. *Mains examination*: The written examination consists of nine papers, two qualifying and seven rankings in nature. The range of questions may vary from just one mark to sixty marks, twenty words to 600 words answers.
3. *Personality test*: 275 marks.

ELIGIBILITY CRITERIA

Nationality
- For the IAS and the IPS, the candidate must be a citizen of India.

Education
- A degree from a Central, State or a Deemed university or equivalent.

Age Limit
- A candidate should be minimum of 21 years and maximum 32 years old as on August 01 of the examination year.
- The upper age limit prescribed above is relaxable for the following candidates:
- *5 years:* Scheduled Caste/Scheduled Tribe (SC/ST)
- *3 years:* Other Backward Classes (OBC)
- *3 years:* Defence Services personnel
- *5 years:* Ex-servicemen including Commissioned Officers and ECOs/SSCOs who have rendered at least 5 years Military Service as on August 01, 2019
- 5 years in the case of ECOs/SSCOs
- *10 years:* Blind, deaf-mute, and orthopedically handicapped persons
- *5 years:* In the case of ECOs/SSCOs who have completed an initial period of assignment of 5 years of Military Service as on 1st August, 2019 and whose assignment has been extended beyond 5 years and in whose case the Ministry of Defence issues a certificate that they can apply for civil employment and that they will be released on 3 months' notice on selection from the date of receipt of offer of appointment.

Number of Attempts

- Restriction on the maximum number of attempts is effective since 1984:
  - *For General Candidates:* 7 attempts (up to 32 years)
  - *Scheduled Caste and Scheduled Tribe Candidates (SC/ST):* No limits (up to 37 years)
  - *Other Backward Classes:* 9 attempts (up to 35 years)
  - *Physically handicapped:* 9 attempts for general and OBC, while unlimited for SC/ST.

Self study for the examination is more important than anything else. "Quality" is more useful than quantity to crack the examination. Several coaching centers and test series for paper solving exist and may be resorted to as per individual preference.

Notes of others should be used very judiciously. It is better to make own notes, because note making, writing and making diagram helps to understand, practice writing and revise better.

DOCTOR AT THE HELM OF ADMINISTRATION

In India, an IAS/IPS officer can really make a difference to the lives of common people even working within the existing system, compared to a doctor. As a doctor, you may have many lucrative earning opportunities along with international endeavors. But those dedicated to the service of motherland would be much happy in pursuing Civil Services. One may earn money abroad, but it is not possible to make even a slight change in the system for the benefit of the people.

Being a Medical Doctor and an IAS officer, you can work for attainment of Universal Access to Equitable, Affordable and Quality health care services. It should be accountable and responsive to people's needs, with effective intersectoral convergent action to address the wider social determinants of health and safeguarding vulnerable health. You can get a chance to safeguard the health of the poor, vulnerable and down privileged. You will be able to move toward a right-based approach to health through entitlements and service guarantees and to strengthen public health systems as a basis for universal access and social protection against the rising costs of health care.

You can build an integrated network of all primary, secondary and a substantial part of tertiary care, providing a continuum from community level to the district hospital, with robust referral linkages to tertiary care and a particular focus on strengthening the Primary Health Care System including outreach services in both rural areas and urban slums. You have to do prioritization of services that address the health of women and children and the prevention and control of communicable and noncommunicable diseases, including locally endemic diseases.

Along with administrative services job duties you will deal with complex public health issues, and will lead the senior colleagues on the planning and delivery of policies and programs that aim to influence the health of groups of people at local, regional and national levels. You will get a chance to plan and lead the evaluation of such programs and provide professional, evidence-based, and ethical advice to guide the commissioning of services, ensuring that they are high-quality, clinically safe, cost effective, and will improve health and well-being and reduce health inequalities across primary care, secondary care, and social care.

If you have a desire for giving back to society, if you wish to bring about a positive change in the lives of people, if you want to bring about a change in the system by being a part of it, after MBBS or MD; then IAS is the perfect opportunity for you to do all this.

As a doctor, you are connected to your patients, their sorrows, their feelings. It gives you insight to connect with the masses at large and solve their problems.

William Osler has said,

"A good Physician treats the disease; the great physician treats the patient who has the disease"

Communication is what is important in medicine as well as in Administration!!

"The Art of Communication is the Language of Leadership"

FURTHER READING

1. Union Public Service Commission (2011). Central Civil Services Examination, 2011 Notice. [online] Available from http://www.upsc.gov.in. [Accessed December, 2018].

CHAPTER 16

Master of Business Administration: New Dimension

Anay Bhalerao

INTRODUCTION

For years, the traditional avenue for a medical student was to become a doctor. However, recently, many of the medical students are opting for nonconventional career choices. One of the enabling routes to do so is to get a degree in *Management Studies*.

Master in Business Administration (MBA) is a lucrative option for many young medical students. It opens up a lot of doors previously thought to be reserved for specialists in different fields, such as Finance, Marketing, Strategy, and Business Consulting. There are also similar specialized courses focused on the healthcare sector, such as Hospital Administration, Pharmaceutical Management, Public Health, and Social Studies. So, if a medical student is looking to do something different, MBA might be a great option (Fig. 16.1).

OPTIONS FOR MBA

As stated earlier, MBA enables a doctor to choose jobs in various sectors. Today, many MBA doctors work successfully in multinational companies that sell things that you use every day as well as boutique venture capital firms that invest in nascent projects.

To understand the opportunities, let us first understand what MBA is all about.

Master in Business Administration is a taught masters course that introduces various aspects of business and teaches the student to tackle

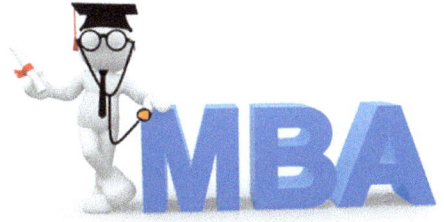

Fig. 16.1: Doctors are opting for an MBA degree nowadays.

various business problems. It is either a degree or a diploma course; however, what matters more is where a student do it from.

You can opt for a full-time MBA program, typically taught for 2 years, or an executive MBA/distant learning MBA program that would be taught for a bit longer. There are 1-year MBA programs available, and a few are equally sought after and are quite rewarding.

In India, the degree awarded is not always MBA. The Indian Institutes of Management (IIMs) offer it as Postgraduate Diploma in Management (PGDM), a few colleges offer it as Postgraduate Diploma in Business Management (PGDBM). Specialized programs have different names as well, such as MBA-Pharmaceutical Management, or Master in Hospital Administration (MHA).

As a rule of the thumb, for a doctor, it makes sense to undergo the full-time course from the top 15 institutes in India. These include the IIMs, XLRI, FMS, MDI, ISB, TISS, among others. The fees for these institutes range from a few thousand to many lakhs, so this should also be taken into consideration.

There are many universities offering the course, however, good companies that offer coveted profiles visit only a few campuses. That said, do not be disheartened if you end up studying at a different college. You never know when you might get lucky.

HOW TO PREPARE FOR AN MBA PROGRAM

Entry to an MBA program is almost always through a rigorous screening process. Applicants are tested for their verbal (read English), Quantitative (read Mathematical), and their analytical skills through a mass screening test. These tests may be paper-based or computer-based.

For India, the nationwide test that one would have to give in order to enter any IIM would be through the Common Admission Test (CAT). In addition, various states hold their own entrance test for the colleges that come under their purview. Different colleges may also hold their own entrance tests, for instance, XLRI admits students via Xavier Aptitude Test.

After clearing the initial MCQ based test, (and at times, an essay), you would be invited for a round of Group Discussion as well as a Personal Interview. These are commonly held on the same day at the same venue for a given college.

Different colleges give different weights to one's performance in academics till the date, one's scores in the screening test, one's scores in the Group discussions, one's personal interviews, job experience, and then decide to admit the students.

For international institutes, the tests may differ and so would the admission procedure. To get into a program in the B-Schools in the USA, you have to give GMAT. ISB Hyderabad is a notable exception in India that accepts GMAT scores for admissions.

Preparing for the Entrance Exams

The entrance tests are not easy, as the skills you are tested on cannot be acquired overnight. Most of the successful students take guidance in the form of coaching for these entrance tests. As with any other exams, solving as many tests as possible, developing your own strategy to maximize your chances in the face of negative marking, and honing your skills would get you through.

If you are even thinking about it, start improving your English today. Read good books about a wide range of topics, as this would come handy during your group discussions and personal interviews. Think of problems in your day-to-day life, and try and solve them through a structured approach. Give ample mock tests and study in groups, it always helps.

CONTENTS OF THE TAUGHT PROGRAM

There are five broad domains for any business—*operations, accounting and finance, marketing and sales, human resources, and strategy*. As a student, you can specialize in one of these, or dabble in all and be a generalist.

Operations refer to how the business "produces" its goods or services. For instance, for a bakery manufacturing bread, operations would entail procuring the wheat, getting it turned to flour, obtaining yeast, mixing the ingredients, proving, baking, and packaging the bread. This also involves deciding how much to manufacture, so that there is enough bread without it going unsold.

Accounting and Finance deal with managing the cash flows—getting money from the customers, using it for operations as well as other activities, and paying the suppliers, in the simplistic sense. It also includes making investments so that the business grows in the future.

The strategy would be to understand what the customer wants, make a "likeable" product, and sell it in such a way that your business objectives are met. For instance, a printer manufacturer may sell the printer at cost, without making much profit, but will ensure that the profit is maximized on the sale of ink.

Marketing would be spreading the word about the product so as to meet the sales targets. The "sales'" function is involved in ensuring that the product is sold according to the business needs.

Human resources would deal with the employees. They would be responsible for maintaining time sheets, planning skill development activities, ensuring that the work environment is fair for everyone.

Naturally, the subjects taught during a typical MBA program would cover all the earlier discussed subjects. Generally speaking, the first year of the MBA program touches these subjects. You end up choosing your specialization by choosing your own subjects during the second year. That said, this may differ from college to college.

The courses are taught in a quite different manner than in the medical school. There are a few subjects, such as Accounting, where you require to learn some rules. However, for most of the rest, it is application of your knowledge in solving business problems. It is usually done using case studies. This is how you learn how companies, big and small, solved the problems they faced in the past.

So, MBA is not a science. It is rather the application of common sense in a very specific manner!

In addition to these, subjects such as Jurisprudence and Business Law, Environmental concerns, Intellectual Property Law, Communication and Negotiation skills could be taught as well. The aim is to enable you to open your own business if you wish to!

WHAT ARE THE OPPORTUNITIES AFTER AN MBA

Now comes the best part. However, before that, you should ask *why* you want to do an MBA?

The MBA is an applied course. It sharpens what is already there within you. However, unlike MBBS, or an MD/MS, MBA does not necessarily guarantee you a job of your liking. The world of business is calculating, and so a company would always assess what benefits it would have in hiring you versus the next candidate in the interview.

MBA does open some doors in healthcare. As a doctor with an MBA, you naturally become an attractive candidate for pharmaceutical companies. You could get into various domains within a pharmaceutical company, including business strategy, Sales and Marketing, or as a Medical Science Liaison.

However, depending on your specialization, you could get a role as an investment banker, a strategist at a fast food company, a medical expert at a Startup, a Business Consultant, or even found your own business.

Today, MBA-doctors, with their sharp analytical and problem-solving skills are doing very well in the space of Banking, Insurance, Investment, Pharmaceuticals, Health-tech start-ups, Blockchain, Hospitals, as well as in the public sector.

As we come toward the end of this chapter, it is important to discuss the pros and cons of opting for this course.

PROS

- As a medical student, you have proved yourself over and over again. It is not easy to gain entrance to the coveted course. However, you took this decision at the age of 18, when you were barely an adult. Naturally, you have some skills previously unexplored, and the unfair systems made you choose between Mathematics and Biology. Most of you were good at both!
- MBA enables you to fulfill all those roles that a medical degree would not allow you to. Granted, MBA is not "necessary" for you to get into those positions, but it does make the process easier.

- You gain entry into the "corporate life". It is lucrative, with early returns, better recognition, an opportunity of working in big diverse teams. It breaks the silos and enables you to succeed if you are good at your job.
- It also lessens the barriers and enables you to work abroad if you so wish.
- It refines a few aspects of your life, like dressing sharply, writing emails, making compelling presentations, public speaking, engaging a boardroom, to name a few.
- You develop a structured approach toward problem-solving. It transcends life as well.
- 5-day week. *Need I say more?*
- And finally, the job is a different kind of stressful, where you are not on call all your life!

THE CONS

- MBA does not automatically make you successful. You have to develop your core competency and excel in every aspect to do good. Two MBA students with the same GPA might not do equally well in the "corporate world".
- In most instances, you are a salaried employee with limited stock options. So, your earning potential is limited *vis a vis* a doctor who has her own practice.
- Some may find the work a bit less meaningful. During the first few years of the job, most of the MBAs end up spending their days on spreadsheets and presentations. It may not be as fulfilling as delivering babies or stitching up the wounds.
- Jobs in healthcare might keep on reminding you what you missed by opting for this course.

PAY SCALE

Depending on the profile offered, the pay scale varies from Rupees 600,000 to Rupees 3,000,000 or more per annum. The annual increment is tied to the performance but the typical trend is to switch jobs in 2–3 years and get a pay hike.

However, as with any other job, salary is only one of the components to consider.

Typically, you can negotiate on benefits such as training program, pension contributions, vacation days, flexible working hours, remote working, and personal insurance coverage to name a few things.

All these may seem flashy and attractive at first, but these are not out of your grasp even if you decide to stay as a doctor.

To sum it up, if you are looking to do something really different, or just looking to become better at handling the business side of your private practice, MBA is a great option for you.

CHAPTER 17

Law Study: An Indispensable and Essential Action (Legum Baccalaureus: Condicio Sine Qua Non)

Manish Y Machave

It is better to prepare and prevent than repair and repent.

INTRODUCTION

The *sacred patient-doctor relationship* is a thing of the past. Common patient complaints pertain to too little time given by doctors. Other concerns are doctors do not listen, do not explain well, show no sympathy and neither understand the patient nor his family.

Why do patients sue is an important perspective. The common issues being "original injury is not enough", perceived lack of caring, altruism—protect others, expose the truth and financial restitution, lack of communication. And importantly over one-third would have opted out of litigation with explanation, appropriate counseling and good communication.

But this fear of law suits has given birth to *defensive medicine*—the use of costly diagnostic efforts of medical treatments for the sole purpose of avoiding potential litigation. Litigation has decreased quality of care as more tests are ordered than medically needed, more specialist referrals than needed, more invasive procedures than needed and more medicines prescribed than needed.

And to add to this is the fact that in cases of litigations, the lawyers and the judges find it extremely difficult to comprehend the conceptual and practical aspects of modern medicines, the comprehensive treatment schedules and the effects of such management on the patient underscoring the various factors which rule them. This affects the decisions in courts; needless to say the duration of time that elapses for such cases. Much to the *anxiety* of the practitioner, justice delayed is justice denied.

Hence in this present scenario it is deemed essential that law be a part of medical education. And till this herculean task is completed it would be more than prudent for all doctors to study law.

BENEFITS OF STUDYING LAW

Medical School and Law School

Most people think of these two demanding courses of study as different and largely unrelated paths. However, the truth is that these fields are increasingly interlinked.

In fact, medical students who also study law are uniquely positioned to navigate the challenges of today's complex healthcare landscape. There exist distinct benefits for a medicine graduate to study law and then pursue his career in medicine.

Studies Offer Enhanced Awareness of Health Policies

While medical students have plenty to learn about anatomy, physiology, biochemistry, and other clinical topics, these things do not exist in a vacuum. Rather, they exist within the very real and very relevant context of national or state healthcare policy.

In order to truly understand the "big picture" of contemporary medicine, a basic understanding of health policy is also required. From issues pertaining to everything from intellectual property to medical malpractice issues, legal factors can make or break a patient's healthcare experience. And while we often think of law as impeding medicine, it can also be used to improve it—with access to the right information.

Law Studies Help Physicians Better Understand and Address Ethical Questions

While medicine can solve many problems, it cannot on its own behave ethically. And while the *Hippocratic Oath* holds physicians to a specific standard of ethical behavior, the underlying issues are far from black and white. Navigating these questions of ethics can be vexing to physicians who lack the tools to manage ethical dilemmas pertaining to issues such as confidentiality, communication and cultural relativism.

Not only have that, but advancements in science, technology and medical research triggered new issues and ethical considerations every day. While these topics are complex, an understanding of the law and ethics can inform the decision-making process for today's physicians.

Law Studies can Support the Doctor-Patient Relationship

Patients are more than their illnesses and conditions, and a doctor's job is far from done when a diagnosis is conferred. In order to truly promote their patients' best interests, physicians must become more than their doctors; they must also become their advocates.

While medical studies enable doctors to treat disease, law studies allow them to do so within the larger context of serving as true patient advocates with the ability to do everything from overcoming barriers to facilitating optimal outcomes.

LAW STUDIES IN THE MEDICAL COLLEGE CURRICULUM

Given our increasing understanding of the reciprocal relationship between law and medicine, it makes sense that more medical colleges should offer cross-disciplinary programs aimed at helping prepare medical and law, students alike for the emerging legal issues of today and tomorrow. In the most basic sense, this involves integrating law studies into the medical school curriculum.

Those looking for more comprehensive educations in medicine and law, meanwhile can take advantage of a growing crop of programs which offer students the opportunity to earn joint degrees in law and medicine.

And while most dual degree graduates do not end up practicing in both professions, they do graduate with a rare and invaluable perspective on healthcare, public policy, and hospital administration. Ultimately, the question of whether this path is right for you lie in your goals.

No one goes to medical school assuming it will be easy. In fact, it is one of the most notoriously difficult academic pathways. Factor in the known rigors of law school, and the merger of the two can be a particularly intensive course of study. However, it's also one which corresponds with profound opportunities— not just for professional advancement, but also in terms of the potential to make a true impact on society.

LAW COURSES AVAILABLE IN INDIA

The law courses available in India are given in Table 17.1.

Table 17.1: Law courses available in India.

Name of the Course	Duration of the course	Advantages	Career options
LLB	3 years	Expertise in law	Litigation, Judiciary, Academics, Civil Services
BA LLB, BBA LLB, B.Com LLB and B.Sc LLB (Hons.)	5 years	Expertise in two streams	Litigation, Judiciary, Academics, Law Firms, Companies, Corporate Counsels Taxation Firms, Law Clerks or Assistants, Regulatory Bodies

Following the national law school model, one can study law as an integrated course of 5 years after passing the senior secondary examination. Bachelor of Laws (LL.B.)—the LL.B. is the most common law degree offered and conferred by Indian universities which has duration of 3 years.

The Bar Council of India has withdrawn the age restriction to take admission in law courses. The students are allowed to take admissions in colleges/universities in LL.B. or LL.M. courses without any age limit.

POSTGRADUATE DIPLOMA IN MEDICOLEGAL SYSTEMS

Postgraduate diploma in medicolegal systems (PGDMLS) is offered as a correspondence course by many deemed universities (Box 17.1). It entitles you to study law related to medicine but does not confer any right to practice as a lawyer.

> **Box 17.1:** Features of postgraduate diploma in medicolegal systems.
> - Duration: 1 Years
> - Level: Diploma after graduation
> - Type: Diploma
> - Eligibility: Graduation

PROPOSAL

A medical school curriculum that addresses the legal context of medical practice should focus on raising awareness of a wide range of subjects and should train students to recognize areas where medical practice and law can come into conflict. Such a curriculum should aim to give medical students concrete tools with which to enter medical practice, with the hope that these tools will help them avoid common legal pitfalls.

A legal medicine curriculum should be broadly divided into three main areas of interest: (1) laws pertaining to the practice of medicine, (2) laws pertaining to ethical conduct, and (3) regulation.

Laws Pertaining to the Practice of Medicine

This area includes topics such as negligence, standards of care, malpractice, acts such as MTP, PCPNDT, BNHR, etc. These subjects are the most relevant to physicians' daily practice and are also the areas where myth often parades as fact.

An examination of the laws that pertain to medical practice should begin by introducing basic concepts from tort law, such as duty to patients, breach of duty, causation of injury, and damages, and then move on to more detailed topics such as risk management and documentation. The legal aspects of the patient-physician relationship should also be covered. In particular, this curriculum should address questions about when a patient-physician relationship legally begins, how to "fire" patients, and how to manage and disclose medical errors.

Laws Pertaining to Ethical Conduct

By "the law of ethics" refers to the jurisprudence behind prominent ethical debates. For example, it is difficult to fully appreciate a physician's role in the debates surrounding end-of-life care without first understanding the legal definitions of death, brain death, assisted suicide, and futility. These areas are deeply rooted in law, and, if they are viewed as purely ethical decisions, the role that courts and legislatures have played in their evolution is overlooked.

Topics that have a clear ethics component are often informed by a wide body of law ranging from legislative statutes and agency regulations to judicial opinions. Though the law does not answer many thorny dilemmas such as how transplantable organs should be distributed, it does provide parameters within which the debate should take place. For example, recent changes to the *Human Organ Transplant Act* have legalized the previously contentious issue of "kidney swapping". While the legalization of such a swap does not eliminate the ethical question of whether such the swap *should* be allowed, it does refocus the debate on how the procedure might be carried out.

Regulation

Regulation cuts the broadest swath in medical jurisprudence, encompassing all areas where the government interacts with and regulates the practice of medicine.

While physicians typically conceive of "the law" mostly in terms of malpractice, the law that they will interact with most during their careers is in the form of regulation. Regulatory agencies from the FDA to the other administrative authorities exercise great power over the practice of medicine and govern physician practices and investment ventures, prescribing guidelines govern how physicians can prescribe controlled substances. Yet health law courses seldom address these topics, even though they are arguably more important than malpractice.

CONCLUSION

Doctor-patient relationship now potentially an adversarial relationship with each patient seen as a potential plaintiff and each question as a possible source of angst.

The current system of medical education fails medical students and trainees by not providing any systematic approach to thinking about the legal issues they will face. Many curricula focus, instead, on ethics, which leaves students without clear guidance on the legal matters they will certainly encounter. While ethics education is important, it should be taught in concert with law.

Students should leave medical school with an appreciation for how the legal system works and how to navigate it. Such awareness may lead to fewer decisions made on the basis of myth and greater comfort in practicing evidence-based medicine over defensive medicine.

And hence it is apt to say: *Legum Baccalaureus-Condicio Sine Qua Non.*

BIBLIOGRAPHY

1. AMA Journal of Ethics. (2008). The Teaching of Law in Medical Education (Shah ND). [online] Available from https://journalofethics.ama-assn.org/article/teaching-law-medical-education/2008-05. [Accessed November, 2018].
2. Healthcare Studies. Masterstudies (Hughes J). [online] Available from https://cdn03.masterstudies.com/img/logo/HealthcareStudies/. [Accessed November, 2018].

CHAPTER 18

MICOG–MRCOG Course

Tushar Kar

Share your knowledge; it is a way to immortality—Dalai Lama

INTRODUCTION

The Indian College of Obstetrics and Gynaecology (ICOG) is the academic wing of Federation of Obstetrics and Gynaecological Society of India (FOGSI), one of the world's largest professional organizations of medical practitioners. ICOG was created to promote education, training, research and spread of knowledge in the field of *obstetrics and gynecology* for students and specialists involved with or interested in women's health care and to address the academic requirements.

Out of numerous activities of ICOG, one important segment is Membership of ICOG (MICOG)-Member of Royal College of Obstetrics and Gynecology, UK (MRCOG)-Part-1 examination. FOGSI-ICOG has combined MICOG with MRCOG Part-1 examination. MRCOG is an international degree, equivalent to postgraduate qualification and recognized by Medical Council of India (MCI) and definitely beneficial for graduates and postgraduates in future. In a year 2 sets of 3 days refresher courses will be conducted approximately 3 months before the examination, i.e. in January and July in a year.

PROCEDURE OF APPLICATION

1. Have FOGSI membership
2. To register with RCOG, first go to www.rcog.org
3. Fill the application form which will be available at RCOG website www.rcog.org in the month of May and November in a year
4. Make a payment of approximately 340 Sterling Pounds to RCOG, UK
5. Send a photocopy of application form which you had sent to RCOG and a demand draft (DD) of ₹ 20,000 in favor of FOGSI along with MBBS registration certificate to FOGSI office, Mumbai toward MICOG fee which includes 3 days refresher course at FOGSI office, Mumbai in the month of January and July of the calendar year.
6. Reputed faculties from RCOG and national faculties will guide you regarding the examination.
7. Once you clear RCOG examination, you will also get a letter of passing MICOG.

MICOG-MRCPI PART 2 EXAMINATION IN INDIA

Federation of Obstetrics and Gynaecological Society of India—ICOG has combined MICOG with MRCPI (Member of Royal College of Physicians of Ireland, Dublin) Part 2 examination. MRCPI is an international degree equivalent as postgraduate qualification and recognized by MCI and definitely beneficial for graduates and postgraduates including diploma holders in future. Each year, one set of examination will take place in September. In a year one set of 2 days refresher course will be conducted before the examination, i.e. in July. Objective Structured Clinical Examination (OSCE) will also be conducted in India in the month of November from 2017; it is twice in a year. Theory examination has been conducted in the month of March and September and OSCE/Clinical examination has been conducted in June and November.

Procedure of Application

1. FOGSI Membership
2. MRCOG Part 1 passing letter
3. To register with MRCPI: First go through www.rcpi.ie
4. Fill the application form which will be available in RCPI website www.rcpi.ie in the month of June/July in a year
5. Payment approximately €710 should be sent to RCPI, Ireland, Dublin
6. Then send a photocopy of application form which you send to RCPI, a DD of ₹ 30,000 in favor of FOGSI with all certificates to FOGSI office, Mumbai toward MICOG fee which includes 2 days refresher course at FOGSI office, Mumbai in the month of July every year.
7. Reputed faculties from RCPI and national faculties will guide you regarding details of examination.
8. Once you clear the RCPI examination both theory and OSCE, you will get a letter of passing of MICOG also.

Since this is an international degree which is equivalent to postgraduate qualification and recognized by MCI, one is able to practice *obstetrics and gynecology* in India and abroad after obtaining the degree.

Index

Page numbers followed by *b* refer to box, *f* refer to figure, and *t* refer to table.

A

Adrenal function 59
American Academy of Family Physicians 106
American Board of Obstetrics and Gynecology 72
American College of Obstetricians and Gynecologists 37, 53
American Society of Clinical Oncology 37
Amniocentesis 55
Andrology 61
    laboratory 60
Anesthesiology 100
Aneuploidy screening 55
Angoff method 92
Anxiety disorder 115
Asherman's syndrome 7
Asia-Pacific Association for Gynecologic Endoscopy 27
Assisted reproductive technology 60
Audit/research related activities 55
Australian Medical Council 99

B

Ball placement 33
Barker's hypothesis 53
Basic electrocautery 33
Biostatics and data management 62
Blastocyst culture 61
Blunt tissue dissection 33
Body dysmorphic disorder 115
Brachytherapy 40
British Society for Gynaecological Endoscopy 25
Burch colposuspension 31

C

Camera control 33
Cell culture 61
Central nervous system, lesions of 73, 76
Chorionic villus sampling 55
Civil services aptitude test 120
Clinical medicine, advanced 104
Clinical psychology and sexology 59
Clitoral hood reduction 112
Coital incontinence 74, 76
Colles' fascia 112
Colposcopy 3
Common admission test 124
Competence progression, annual review of 88
Complete da Vinci technology
    in-service with da Vinci representative 32
    online
        assessment 32
        training 32
    skills drills session 33
Complete live standard case observation 32
Completion of training, certificate of 87
Complex da Vinci procedure
    observation 34
    video review 34
Controlled ovarian stimulation 60
Cosmetic gynecology 3, 110, 115
    opportunities in 115
    surgical procedures in 111
Cryopreservation 61
    principles of 61
Culture media 61

D

da Vinci surgery
  procedure 32, 33
  webinar 34
da Vinci surgical system 32
da Vinci technology 32
  skills drills 32
  training 32
da Vinci training
  certificate, sample of 34*f*
  passport technology training pathway 32
Delivery, management of 89
Designer laser vaginoplasty 111, 113
Detrusor overactivity 75
Diverticula 73, 76

E

Early pregnancy
  after ART treatment
    monitoring of 62
    treatment of 62
  ultrasound 55
Ebel's method 90
E-learning 90
Electronic
  residency application service 50
  urodynamics studies 74
Embryo
  donation 62
  freezing 61
  hatching 61
  transfer 61, 62
Embryology 60
  lab 59, 60
    quality control and maintenance 61
Emotional and behavioral disorders 73, 76
Endocrine disturbances 59
Endocrinology 59
Endometrial receptivity assay 61
Endometriosis 7, 31
Endometrium, transcervical resection of 7
Endoscopic surgery 60
European Academy of Gynaecological Surgery 25
European Board and College of Obstetrics and Gynecology 24
European Society of Aesthetic Gynecology 115
European Society of Gynaecological Endoscopy 24, 29
European Urogynecological Association 72
Evidence-based medicine, principles of 74

F

Family medicine 100
Family planning 85, 108
  program 85
Fecal incontinence 73
Federation of Obstetrics and Gynaecological Society of India 133, 134
Federation of State Medical Boards 100
Fellowship 108
  admission test 57
  clinical 27
  programs in India, map of 49*f*
Female genital plastic surgery 111
Female infertility
  diagnosis of 60
  management of 60
Female pelvic medicine 71
  and reconstructive surgery 108
Female reproductive system 59
Fertility preservation 62
Fertilization 60
  abnormal 61
  normal 61
Fetal anomalies, targeted imaging for 55
Fetal autopsies 55
Fetal medicine 42, 55
  and perinatology 59
  fellowships 50
  foundation 50
Fetal origin of adult disease 53
Fibroids 7, 31
Fluid management 77
Foreign medical graduates, education commission for 100
Fourth arm control 33
Freezing techniques 61
Frenkel hypothesis 53

Index **137**

G

Gametes
  storage of 61
  use of 61
Gametogenesis 60
Genetic 60
  history and counseling 61
German Academy of Obstetrics and
    Gynecology 29
German Association of Gynecological
    Endoscopy 29
German Society of Gynecological
    Endoscopy 26
German Society of Urogynecology 72
Grafenberg spot 113
Growth scans 55
Gynecologic malignancies 41
Gynecologic oncologist, role of 36
Gynecologic oncology 108
  fellowship 41
  programs 39
Gynecological endoscopic surgeries,
    advanced 28
Gynecological endoscopy
  task force for accreditation of 27
  training 6
Gynecological oncology 31, 36

H

Hands-on live surgery 28
Hands-on practice 27
Health professional shortage area 107
High-risk pregnancy 54
  and perinatology 53
Hormone
  autocrine 59
  deficiency states 76
  on pelvic floor 74
Human Organ Transplant Act 132
Human reproduction 59
Hymenoplasty 112
Hyperandrogenic states 60
Hypothalamic-pituitary-ovarian hormones
    59
Hysterectomy
  benign 31
  laparoscopic 7

Hysteropexy 31
Hysteroscopic surgeries 7
Hysteroscopy 2, 60

I

In vitro fertilization 60, 64
Indian College of Obstetrics and
    Gynaecology 133
Indian Corporate Law Service 117
Indian Council of Medical Research 36
Indian Defence Accounts Service 117
Indian Defence Estates Service 118
Indian Federal Law Enforcement Agencies
    119
Indian Foreign Service 117, 118
Indian Forest Service 117
Indian Information Service 118
Indian Ordnance Factories Service 118
Indian Police Service 117, 119
Indian Post and Telecommunication
    Accounts and Finance Service 117
Indian Postal Service 118
Indian Railway Accounts Service 118
Indian Railway Personnel Service 118
Indian Railway Traffic Service 118
Indian Revenue Service 117, 118
Indian Trade Service 118
Infertility 60
  management, ethical and medicolegal
      aspects of 62
Insemination 61
Internal medicine 100
International Fellowship Programs, map
    of 50*f*
International horizon 85
International Society of
    Cosmetogynecology 115
International Society of Gynecological
    Endoscopy 26
International Urogynecological
    Association 72
Interstitial cystitis 73
Intracytoplasmic sperm injection 60
  techniques of 61
Intrauterine insemination 60
Italian School of Endoscopy 28

K

Kiel School of Gynecological Endoscopy 26
Knot tying 33

L

Labia majora
    augmentation 112, 113
    laser reduction of 113
    liposculpturing of 113
    reduction 112
Labia minora thickness, reduction of 113
Labiaplasty 112
Labor, management of 89
Laparoscopic Institute for Gynecology and Oncology 25
Laparoscopic training centers outside India, list of 24
Laparoscopy 2, 24, 28, 60
    operative 62
    process of 2f
Laser labiaplasty 112
Laser vaginal
    rejuvenation 111, 113
    tightening 113
Laser vulval lightening 114
Law courses available in India 130t
Law study 128
    in medical college curriculum 129
List of Indian College of Obstetricians and Gynecology recognized centers for certificate course in reproductive medicine 65
Lower bowel urinary tract 76
Lower gastrointestinal tract
    fistulae 76
    function, disorders of 76
Lower intestinal tract, disorders of 73
Lower urinary and intestinal tract
    fistulae 73
    function 73
Lower urinary tract 76
    and pelvis
        anatomy of 77
        function of 77

M

Majora reduction 112
Male infertility
    diagnosis of 60
    management of 60
Male reproductive system 59
Maternal and child health 4
Maternal fetal medicine 3, 42, 49, 50, 53, 56, 108
    certification in 51
Medical Council of Canada Qualifying Examination 99
Medical Council of India 57, 99
Medical School and Law School 128
Medical statistics 62
Medical teaching 81
Medicolegal and ethical aspect 62
Medicolegal cases 3
Medicolegal Committee 5
Mentors' evaluation 27
Minimal access surgery 108
    diploma 28
    training 27
Minimal hysteroscopy surgeries 28
Minimal invasive surgery 24, 28, 30, 39
Minimal invasive surgical
    procedures 30
    techniques 24
Minimal invasive therapy 27
Mons pubis, liposculpturing of 113
Mons reduction 112
MRCOG exam, tips for 91b, 95b, 98b

N

National Board of Examinations 53, 54, 57
National Board of Medical Education 100
National Eligibility Cum Entrance Test 36, 58
National Health Mission 83
National Resident Matching Program 104
National Training Number 87
Neurology 77
Nonelectronic urodynamics studies 74
Nuchal translucency 54

O

Obstetric anal sphincter injury 73, 76
Obstetrical and gynecological ultrasound, certification in 51
Oocyte
  donation 62
  freezing 61
  identification and grading 61
Orthopedic surgery 100
Ovarian
  hormones 59
  hyperstimulation syndrome 61
  tumors, benign 7
Overactive bladder syndrome 73, 75
Ovulation 59
  induction 60
  monitoring of 60
Ovum pick-up 61

P

Painful bladder syndrome 73, 76
Paracrine hormones 59
Pediatric labial hypertrophy 110
Pelvic floor 73, 76
  defects 7
  disorders 73, 74
  function 73
  trauma, childbirth related 73
Pelvic organ prolapse 73, 76
Pelvic pain 76
  syndrome 73
Pelvic problems 89
Pelvic surgery, effects of 76
Personality test 120
Pharmacological therapies 77
Platelet rich plasma 112, 113
Polycystic ovary syndrome 60
Port placement, instrument control 33
Postgraduate diploma in medicolegal systems 130
  features of 131b
Pregnancy
  care, inverted pyramid of 53
  multiple 61
Preimplantation genetic diagnosis 61
  screening 61
Prenatal invasive diagnostic procedures 55

Professional and linguistic assessment board test 99
Proximal tubal cannulation 7
Psychiatry 100
Psychosis 115
Puberty disorders, normal 60
Public health sector and family planning 80

R

Reconstructive pelvic surgery 71
Rectal prolapse 73
Reproductive
  endocrinology 59
    and infertility 108
  genetics, basics of 61
  immunology 60
  medicine 3, 59
    and surgery 57, 64, 68t
    application of 4f
  ultrasonography in 60
Revirgination procedure 112
Robotic gynecology 31
Robotic operating system 30f
Robotic surgery 3, 30, 108
  process of 3f
Royal College of Obstetricians and Gynaecologists 28, 51, 53, 72, 87, 87f
  membership of 50, 87
Royal College of Physicians of Ireland, member of 134

S

Sacrocolpopexy 31
Saudi Medical Licensing Examination 99
Science and Engineering Research Board 36
Semen
  analysis 60, 62
  freezing 61
Septal resection 7
Sex development, disorders of 60
Sexual and reproductive health 89
Sexual dysfunction 74
Sexually transmitted diseases 74, 76
Sir Nicolaides hypothesis 53

Skills
  drills 32
  simulator 32
Slow freeze techniques/vitrification 61
Society of Laparoscopy Surgeon 26
Society of Obstetricians and
      Gynaecologists 72
Spatial control 33
Sperm
  donation 62
  function tests 60
  wash procedures 62
Studying law, benefits of 128
Submucus fibroid removal 7
Surgeon lecture program 34
Surgery
  effects of 73
  laparoscopic 7
Surgical video editing 27
Surrogacy 62

T

Teratogenesis, fuel mediated 53
Testicular/epididymal sperms, processing
      samples of 60
Testis
  PESA 62
  TESA 62
  TESE 62
Third party reproduction 62
Thyroid 59
Tissue
  cutting 33
  retraction 33
Training centers, details of 7
Training programs 37
  aims and objectives of 39
Tubal recanalization procedures 62
Tubal surgeries 7

U

Union Public Service Commission 80, 81,
    117
United States Medical Licensing
    Examination 4, 99
  Course, three-step process of 102*f*

University Hospital for Gynecology 29
University recognized fellowship, list of
    69*t*
Urethral lesions 73, 76
Urinary
  disorders in
    childhood 73, 76
    pregnancy 73, 76
  incontinence types assessment 73
  problems 74, 76
  retention 73, 75
  tract infection 73
Urodynamic stress incontinence 75
Urogynecology 72, 73
  condition, conservative management of
    77
  fellowship 71
  laparoscopic 77
Urology 59
USMLE
  and future prospects 99
  exam details 105
  steps 102
Uterine bleeding, abnormal 60

V

Vaginal rejuvenation 112, 113
Vaginal skin lightening 114
Vaginal tightening, nonsurgical 111*f*
Vessel dissection 33
Voiding disorders 75
Voiding dysfunction 73
Vulvar disorders 74
Vulvar structures, suprapubic lift of 113
V-wedge technique, modified 111

W

Wedge resection 112
World and Kaplan pretest 100
W-plasty 112

X

Xavier aptitude test 124

EU GSPR Authorised Reprsentative
Logos Europe, 9 rue Nicolas Poussin
1700, La Rochelle, France
Phone: +33 (0) 6 67 93 73 78
E-mail: contact@logoseurope.eu

www.ingramcontent.com/pod-product-compliance
Ingram Content Group UK Ltd.
Pitfield, Milton Keynes, MK11 3LW, UK
UKHW050428150426
5217IPUK00019B/1294